PSYCHOLOGY
for
GRADUATE NURSES

(BSc Nursing, Post Basic Nursing)

PSYCHOLOGY *for* GRADUATE NURSES

(BSc Nursing, Post Basic Nursing)

RAJESH G KONNUR
MPhil (N) PhD MBA PGDGC PGDCA
Professor cum Vice Principal
SGRD College of Nursing Vallah
Amritsar, Punjab, India

Foreword

Dr Laxmi Rana

JAYPEE BROTHERS MEDICAL PUBLISHERS (P) LTD

New Delhi • Panama City • London • Dhaka • Kathmandu

Jaypee Brothers Medical Publishers (P) Ltd

Headquarter

Jaypee Brothers Medical Publishers (P) Ltd
4838/24, Ansari Road, Daryaganj
New Delhi 110 002, India
Phone: +91-11-43574357
Fax: +91-11-43574314
Email: jaypee@jaypeebrothers.com

Overseas Offices

J.P. Medical Ltd.
83 Victoria Street, London
SW1H 0HW (UK)
Phone: +44-2031708910
Fax: +02-03-0086180
Email: info@jpmedpub.com

Jaypee-Highlights Medical Publishers Inc.
City of Knowledge, Bld. 237, Clayton
Panama City, Panama
Phone: + 507-301-0496
Fax: + 507-301-0499
Email: cservice@jphmedical.com

Jaypee Brothers Medical Publishers (P) Ltd
17/1-B Babar Road, Block-B, Shaymali
Mohammadpur, Dhaka-1207
Bangladesh
Mobile: +08801912003485
Email: jaypeedhaka@gmail.com

Jaypee Brothers Medical Publishers (P) Ltd
Shorakhute, Kathmandu
Nepal
Phone: +00977-9841528578
Email: jaypee.nepal@gmail.com

Website: www.jaypeebrothers.com
Website: www.jaypeedigital.com

Inquiries for bulk sales may be solicited at: jaypee@jaypeebrothers.com

Psychology for Graduate Nurses (BSc Nursing, Post Basic Nursing)

First Edition: **2013**

ISBN 978-93-5090-203-5

Printed at: Rajkamal Electric Press, Plot No. 2, Phase-IV, Kundli, Haryana.

Dedicated to

My grandfather late Shri KN Konnur
a great visionary and educationist

Foreword

It gives me a great pleasure to write the Foreword for the book "Psychology for Graduate Nurses" by Dr Rajesh Konnur. The book is comprehensive. It covers all the components of human psychology such as attention, perception, motivation related learning and thinking. It covers developmental psychology, personality and other related areas of adjustment. The content also focuses on psychological problem and various test related to mental health and hygiene.

I think the efforts of the author are appreciable. I know Rajesh Konnur personally. He is hard-working, enthusiastic and challenging. I congratulate him for his exhaustive strive for the remarkable achievement.

I am confident that the book will be of great value for the nurse educators, students and clinicians who are interested in the human psychology and educational psychology as well as mental health.

Laxmi Rana
PhD
Principal
Jaya College of Nursing
Gwalior, Madhya Pradesh, India

PREFACE

This book is designed for those who seek a comprehensive view of the profession of psychology in nursing, readers will find a broad, detailed, in-depth information about the general concepts of psychology.

The contents of the book are prepared according to the syllabus of Indian Nursing Council to enable the nursing students to use it as a textbook for psychology. It will also helpful the nurse educators to teach and prepare students for their practical application. It can also be referred by other allied health professionals.

The whole book is divided into units. Each Unit provides introduction, contents, summary and review questions for self evaluation. At the end of the book a form is attached to get readers feedback. Readers can communicate for further improvement.

I am very thankful to all who contributed to bring this book.

A special acknowledgment is to Shri Jitendar P Vij (Group Chairman) M/s Jaypee Brothers Medical Publishers Pvt Ltd. New Delhi, India and distributors, New Delhi for taking keen interest in publishing this book.

Rajesh G Konnur

CONTENTS

Chapter 1

Introduction to Psychology

INTRODUCTION

Today, we all are in a stressful world, facing many challenges against us. To overcome these challenges, we have to know the root cause and its effects. The study which deals with aspects of life is psychology.

HISTORY AND ORIGIN OF PSYCHOLOGY

Psychology was born of two parents, philosophy and physiology. Psychology has rich roots dating back to the views of Greek philosophers, such as Socrates, Plato and Aristotle, on the nature of mind, the soul, the body, and of human experience. One of the earliest debates about human psychology is still raging today, the question of whether human capabilities are inborn or acquired through experience. The nativist view is that human beings enter the world with an inborn store of knowledge and understands of reality. Early philosophers believed that the knowledge and understanding could be accessed through careful reasoning and introspection. Descartes, in the 17th century, supported the nativist view by arguing that some ideas (such as God, the self perfection, and infinity) are innate at birth. Descartes is also notable for his conception of the body as a machine that can be studied as other machines are studied. This is the root of modern day information processing perspectives on the mind.

The empiricist views that knowledge is acquired through experience and interactions with the world. This view is strongly associated with 17th century English philosopher John Locke. According to Locke, humans are born with tabula rasa, or with a blank state, onto which experience in the world writes all knowledge and understanding. This perspective gave birth to associationist psychology. The associationists denied inborn ideas or capabilities of the mind. Instead, they argued that the mind was filled with ideas that entered by way of the senses and then become associated through such principles as similarity, contrast, and contiguities. Current research findings on memory and learning is related to earlier association theory.

These days, the debate between nativism and empiricism is referred to as the nature versus nurture debate. Although some psychologists would still argue that human thought and behavior is the result primarily of biology or primarily of experience, most psychologists take a more integrated approach, acknowledging that biological processes (such as heredity or processes in the brain) affect thoughts and behavior, but experience also leaves its mark on thoughts and behavior.

For clear understanding, the development of psychology can be divided as below:

1. The early age of prescientific psychology.
2. The modern age of scientific psychology.
3. Contemporary psychology.

Early Age of Prescientific Psychology

In the earliest period of the history of psychology, theorists were answered quite unscientifically on the basis of superstition and speculations as follows.

It was believed that a person's behavior was the result of his fate which was bound to be influenced by the movements of the planets. Besides the role of planets, demons, spirit, ghosts and other supernatural forces were held responsible for human actions. The causes and forms of human behavior were being located outside the human being.

Modern Age of Scientific Psychology

In the 19th century with the influence of research in the field of physics, chemistry, biology, medicine, and technology and other natural sciences, it was felt that human behavior should be tested. While explaining how the study of human behavior should be performed, the researchers presented their views in different systems or schools of psychology. These are presented as follows.

Structuralism

Wilbelm Wundt (The father of experimental psychology) a German physician who established the world's first psychological laboratory at Leipzing in 1879. His experiments focused on conscious experience involving one's thoughts, feelings, sensations, perceptions and ideas. He experimented on the speed of thought and applied scientific methodology of physiologists. He built a device called a thought meter. As he emphasized on the analysis of the components of consciousness by using the art of introspection or self observation; the approach to psychology was named as structuralism.

Functionalism

It was the first American approach to the study of psychology. John Dewey (1859–1952) and William James (1842–1910) were propagated functionalism. The pioneers recognized the mind to be a recent development in the evolutionary process, the function of which was to aid man's adjustment to his environment. The theorists further emphasized that habits were nothing but the functions of the nervous system.

Behaviorism and S-R psychology

American Psychologist, John B Watson (1878–1958), developed behaviorism. He concluded that the whole idea of consciousness is absurd. Consciousness cannot be proved by any scientific test, cannot be seen, nor touched, nor exhibited in a test tube. Even if exists it cannot be studied in a scientific way; because it is subjected to private inspection. Therefore, if we intend to make psychology a science of behavior, we have to discard altogether not only the concept of consciousness but also all the mentalistic notion like soul, mind, mental life, images and ideas, dreams or the actions of a supposed unconscious mind. For this reason, behaviorism was also referred to as black box psychology because its earlier proponents considered the mind to be like a mysterious black box whose contents could never be examined objectively.

A branch of behaviorism known as S-R psychology (stimulus –response) remains an important force in modern psychology. It states that our behavior is the product of our immediate environment and of our past experiences. S-R psychologists have shown that the associations we experience—the pleasant or unpleasant consequences following our actions and our observations of the actions of those around us, called social learning, often determine our responses. Through behavioral technology, problems such as aggression, phobias, shyness and poor study habits can be corrected.

GESTALT PSYCHOLOGY

Gestalt psychology was born against structuralism and functionalism in Germany. The most prominent members of this school were Max Wertheimer (1880–1943). Wolfgang Kobler (1887–1967), Kurt Kofflea (1886–1941) and Kurt Lewin (1890–1947).

The word Gestalt is a German noun. In English it is termed as "configuration" or more simply, which means "an organized whole in contrast to a collection of parts". It is opposed to the atomistic and molecular approach to behavior. Gestalt theorists views an individual perceives the thing as a whole and not as a mere collection of its constituents or elements. The meaning of sensation or perception is always related to the total situation. Perception involves a problem of organization. A thing is perceived as a relationship within a field which includes the thing, the viewer and a complex background incorporating the viewer's purpose and previous experiences. Gestalt theorists asserted that there lies definitely a sort of organization between the stimulus and response which helps in forming a new gestalt (an organized whole).

For example: when looking at watch, what is seen is a watch? It may be that a watch consists of color, brightness and a form but when perceived by the mind all these components become a pattern, or a gestalt. The propognists of this theory, further claim that when the components of a thing are brought together by the mind something new, even more valuable and comprehensive than the original components may emerge consolidating the statement that the "whole is different from the sum of its parts". As a result, the human behavior is characterized as an intelligent behavior rather than simple stimulus-response mechanization. An individual perceives the situation as a whole and after seeing and evaluating the different relationships in relation to the available environment takes the proper decision in an intelligent way: although quite often all of a sudden. Gestalt psychology used the term "insight" to describe this type of human behavior and summarized the behavioral processes as:

a. Perception of the situation as a whole
b. Seeing and judging the relationships between various factors involved in the situation
c. Taking an immediate decision and behaving accordingly.

Gestalt psychology opposed traditional psychology and deplored the "brick and mortar" concept of structuralism—meaning elements "bricks" bound by association "mortar"—and were equally dissatisfied with the S-R conditioning or machine like explanation of human behavior.

The Gestalt psychology is still prevalent throughout modern psychology. It is now well appreciated that many experiences must be analyzed and understood as whole entities and cannot necessarily be broken into constituent parts.

PSYCHOANALYSIS/ PSYCHOANALYTIC THEORY

Psychoanalytic theory was developed by a Viennese physician, Sigmund Freud (1856–1939). The theory comprises the following views.

Unconscious

Freud claimed that the mind is like an iceberg in that most of it is hidden beneath the surface. The conscious part occupies only one-tenth portion of the total mental life. In fact, there is an even stronger force-underlying behavior, the unconscious. This vast part of the mental life of human beings remains hidden and usually inaccessible. It contains all the repressed wishes, desires, feelings, drives and motives—many of which relate to sex and aggression. This hidden treasure of the human mental life is responsible for most of his behavior. The key to the solution of most behavioral problems lies in bringing the unconscious to the conscious level.

Psychoanalytic Method

Sigmund Freud emphasized more importance to the long forgotten or repressed childhood experiences for the determination of problems of adulthood. His method is known as psychoanalytical method for the solution of behavioral problems. It involves the process of analyzing the underlying unconscious behavior. Freud advocated the following techniques:

Free Association

In this technique the affected individual is made to lie on a couch and say anything that comes into his or her mind, no matter how trivial or ridiculous it may seem.

Dream Analysis

Sigmund Freud argues that dreams are disguised representations of repressed desires, which appear in symbolic form. This is known as the dream's latent content. In this view, the purpose of dreams is to provide unconscious gratification, so that certain desires can be satisfied and thus, will not intrude into the sleeper's life when he is awake. Only the surface or manifest content of dreams is open to straight forward observation.

The analysis of these dreams can reveal the unconscious mind and thus, may take to the roots of the abnormalities.

Analysis of the Daily Psychopathology

The repressed desires or experiences lying in the unconscious can also be revealed through day to day psychopathology in terms of the slips of the tongue, slips of the pen, forgotten names and forgotten appointments, lost gifts and mislaid possessions.

Structure of Personality

Freud divided his topographic model of personality into three major systems that interact to govern human behavior, the Id, the Ego and the Superego:

Id: The Id is the most primitive part of the personality, from which the ego and the superego later develop. It is present in the newborn infant and consists of the basic biological impulses (or drives): the need to eat, to drink, to eliminate wastes, to avoid pain and to gain sexual (sensual) pleasure. Freud believed that aggression is also a basic biological drive. The Id seeks immediate gratification of these impulses. The Id operates on the pleasure principle: It endeavors to obtain pleasure and to avoid pain, regardless of the external circumstances.

Ego: It develops out of the Id and acts as an intermediary between the forces, i.e. instinctual demands of the realities of the external world and ethical, moral demands of the superego. The ego acts on reality principle. The gratification of impulses must be delayed until the situation is appropriate. It is essentially the executive part of the personality. It decides what actions are appropriate and which Id impulses will be satisfied and in what manner. The ego mediates among the demands of the Id, the realities of the world and the demands of the superego.

Superego: It is the ethical-moral aspect of the psyche. It judges whether actions are right or wrong. The superego is the internalized representation of the values and morals of society and comprises the individual's conscience as well as his or her image of

Frued compared the human mind with an Iceberg

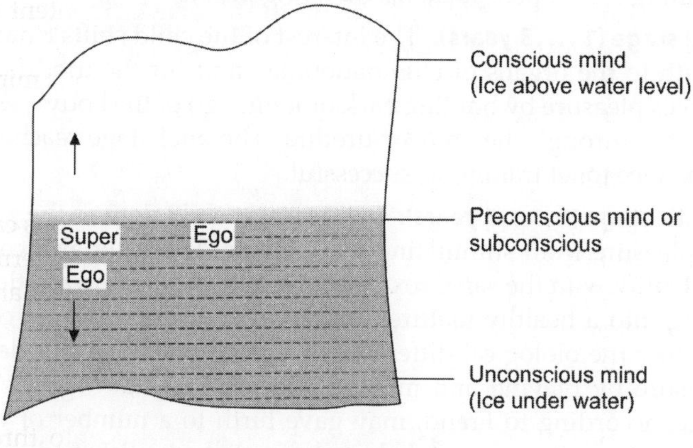

(Diagram explaining the level of consciousness)

Fig. 1.1: Freud's structural model of mind (Ref by Dr Kasturi Psychaitric Nursing)

the morally ideal person (ego ideal). The superego develops in response to parental rewards and punishments.

All behavior, according to Freud, can be understood in terms of the dynamic equilibrium among Id, ego and superego. The Id demands to satisfy its needs and appetites while the ego tries both, to control the Id in terms of reality and to appease the superego. The well adjusted individual is governed by the ego, the anxious neurotic by guilt from his superego; the psychopathic by his Id. The aim of psychoanalysis is to restore the balance, where Id was 'there shall ego be'.

Psychosexual Development

In Freud's view, child development is an important predictor of later adult personality. During development, each person passes through five psychosexual stages. Sex is the life urge or fundamental motive in life. All physical pleasures arising from any of the organs or any of the functions are ultimately sexual in nature. Sexuality is not the characteristic of only the adolescent. Children from the very beginning also have sexual desires. This, he quoted as infantile sexuality.

Oral stage (Birth ..... 1 year): In this stage, mouth represents the first sex organ for providing pleasure to the child. The beginning is made with the pleasure received from the mother's nipple or the "bottle", thereafter; it is used to derive pleasure by putting anything ...... pen, stick, his own fingers, etc.

Anal stage (1 .... 3 years): The interest of the child shifts from the mouth to the organs of elimination, i.e. anus or the urethra. He derives pleasure by holding back or letting go of the body's waste material through the anus or urethra. The anal stage reaches its peak once toilet training is successful.

Phallic stage (4 ..... 6 years): In this stage, child derives the greatest pleasure from stimulating the genitals. The child also comes to identify with the same sex parent, a critical step, toward developing into a healthy mature adult. At this stage, children come to know the biological differences between the sexes and derive pleasure by playing and manipulating the genital organs. This stage, according to Freud, may gave birth to a number of complexes like deprivation and electra complexes in girls and castration and oedipus complexes in boys. Deprivation is the result of the feeling generated into the minds of the little girls that they have been deprived of the male organs by their mothers. Castration complex is generated in boys through the fear of being deprived of the male organs certainly as a result of the organ if they did not leave the habit of playing with it. Oedipus and electra are the results of the sexual attraction or pleasure the children receive in the company of the opposite sex parent. In case, the like sex parent frustrates the desire, expresses his or her resentment and is not friendly to the boy or girl, the child may be likely to develop oedipus or electra complex by loving more the opposite sex parent and rather hating the like sex parent.

Latency stage (6 years ..... puberty): At this stage, boys and girls prefer to be in the company of their own sex and even neglect or hate the members of opposite sex.

Genital stage (Puberty ... adulthood): In this stage, heterosexual desire awakens and attraction toward opposite sex. According to Freud, if transition does not go smoothly, it gives rise to developmental problems. Fixation may occur at any stage. For example, if a child's Id does not receive enough satisfaction during the oral stage, the child may be reluctant to leave that stage until he feels fully satisfied. Fixation may be positive or negative.

As an example of fixation, an individual might remain immature in his social relations and engage excessively in oral activities, such as eating, talking and smoking. Such behavior in adolescence might result from negative or positive fixation during the oral stage. Any fixation can lead to problems. If a child's Id was not satisfied during toilet training, because of the demands made by parents, the child may get satisfaction through undue retention-an anal fixation. Freud believed that such an anal retentive personality would be expressed as selfishness, stinginess, lying, etc.

Recent developments in contemporary psychology: The theorists of different schools of psychology the structuralism, functionalism, behaviorism, gestaltitism and psychoanalysis focuses on the weaknesses of other schools. Today's psychology witnesses an electic approach in dealing with human behavior by accepting the fact that the different view points help in one way or other in studying the complex human behavior by throwing light on other aspects of life.

Humanistic psychology: This uses humanism in psychology. The theorists like Abraham Maslow, Rollo May, Arthur Combs, Caviar Rogers, Gordon All posts have contributed towards its inception and growth. This gives more value to human being by not considering him merely as a sophisticated machine or victim of conflict between Id and ego. It considers him as a purposeful being; capable of adapting himself to his environment and choosing his own course of action toward self-actualization.

Transpersonal Psychology

This is one of the latest approaches in contemporary psychology. The contribution of Abraham Maslow in terms of realization of self, one's fullest potential considered the corner-stone of this school of psychology. It focuses on attention on the study of personal experiences that seem to transcend ordinary existence. In other terms, what we think and how we do feel in our altered states of awareness may be focus area of the transpersonal psychology. These states may be reached during severe stress and distress or in the moments of great excitement and happiness. They may be aroused during periods of sleep or deep concentration. Practically, they may be induced with the help of the influences brought about by specific drugs, religious practices, yoga and transcendental meditation, etc.

Cognitive Psychology

Cognition refers to thinking, remembering and perceiving. Wilhelm Wundt, Donald Broadbent, is the main theorists of cognitive psychology. It is the result of intellectualism which believes in higher cognitive abilities and capacities of human being for his adaptation to his environment and struggle for perfection. It studies all about man's thinking, memory, language, development, perception, imagery and other higher mental processes in order to study the mental functions like insight, creativity and problem solving. Cognitive psychologists are totally opposed to the stimulus response approach of the behaviorists. They maintain that there is something more to learning and behaving man just single responses to stimuli. The human mind does not accept information from its environment in exactly the same form and style as it is conveyed to him. The conveyed information is compared with the already stored information in the mind; it is then analyzed and often enlarged upon, for giving it a quite new form. Then, it is subjected to interpretation and use or storage according to the needs of the situation.

The newer contribution to psychology by Herbert Simon who research on how psychological phenomena could be simulated using the computer. Man is a information-processing system. The human being viewed as a processor of information. The senses provide an input channel for information, mental operations are applied to the input; the transformed input creates a mental structure interacts with others in memory to generate a response.

Another major change in modern psychology is the development of modern linguistics. The linguistics theorizes about the mental structures required to comprehend and to speak a language. The pioneering work was done by Noam Chomsky. A development in the field of psycholinguistics provides the first significant psychological analysis of language.

Definition of Psychology

The word "psychology" is derived from two Greek words, 'psycho' and 'logos; psyche means 'soul' and 'logos' means 'the study of'. Hence, the earliest definition of psychology was that it is the study of 'soul' or 'spirit'. The word 'soul' was used rather very vaguely and there were many interpretations that could be given to it. Hence later on, the term 'mind' replaced 'soul'. Thereafter, psychology was regarded as the study of an individual's mind or mental processes. This definition was given up as unsatisfactory because the mind as an object does not exist; what exists is only the brain. In other words, the mind is not a thing but a 'function'. It is difficult to study the mind apart from what it does. In other terms, we can study it only when it functions or operates in human, behavior or activities.

Psychology has also been defined as the science of consciousness. Wilhelm Wundt (1832–1920) defined psychology as the science of immediate experience with consciousness being the main subject matter.

Titchner (1867–1927), the leader of the structuralists defines psychology as the science of conscious experience which is dependent upon the experiencing person.

Watson (1878–1958) defines psychology as a science and as a science it is to limit itself to the study and analysis of publicly observable elements such as the behavior of the subject rather than subjective matters like his private mental states.

Meaning of Science and Behavior

Science has been defined as "systematic study of knowledge" concerning the relationship between the cause and effect of a particular phenomena. In order to collect the scientific data and systematized material, science employs various kinds of methods of enquiry such as observation, classification, formulation of hypothesis, analysis and interpretation of evidence, etc. It also organizes and develops our knowledge of the world, we live on. Psychology too aims at same thing. It uses scientific methods to study human behavior. It also helps us to understand, control and predict human behavior.

Psychology is a positive or natural science, not a normative one. It describes the facts of human behavior and its laws as they are rather than as they ought to be. Ethics is a normative science because it deals with behavior as it should be. Logic is a normative science because it deals with how we should think. In positive sciences, we merely describe behavior as we discover or find it without evaluating it, without saying whether it is good or bad; but in normative sciences, we evaluate behavior and thus, attempt to influence or improve the behavior of others.

Behavior includes all types of human activities – motor activities like walking and speaking; cognitive activities such as perceiving, remembering, thinking or reasoning; and emotional activities like feeling happy, sad, angry, or afraid. It is both bodily and mental. Mental behavior such as thinking, reasoning, imaging, problem solving, analyzing as "mental experiences or processes". Bodily behavior refers to the movements and action of the body in response to a situation.

Our behavior is a matter of growth and development from infancy to old age. At each stage, our behavior shows certain unique characteristic features. Psychology as a science of behavior studies these characteristic features, and compares and contrasts them from each stage to another. It also studies the differences in behavior, between an individual and another in the same stage of development, between man and animal, between a normal person and psychologically deviated or abnormal person.

SCOPE OF PSYCHOLOGY

Scope includes the limits, branches, topics and subject matter. The field of operation and application of the subject of psychology is too vast. It studies, describes, explains, explores and does scientific findings in behavior of the living organisms. Behavior includes all types of life activities and experiences, which includes cognitive, conative, implicit, or explicit, conscious, unconscious/subconscious, affective of a living entity. The term living organisms includes all the living creatures created by the almighty on this earth and space irrespective of their species, caste, color, age, and sex, mental or physical state. Thus, it studies all aspects of normalcy, abnormal, children, adult, criminals, consumers and producers belonging to different walkers of human life—all are studied under the umbrella of psychology. It also studies the behavior of the animals, insects, birds and even plant life. Thus, it studies all aspects of human life activities.

Branches/Areas of Specialization

For convenience, the subject of psychology is divided into pure psychology and applied psychology.

Pure Psychology

It provides the framework and theory. Its contents deal with the formulation of psychological principles and theories. Pure psychology suggests various methods and techniques for the assessment, analysis, and improvement of behavior.

Applied Psychology

It is the use of pure psychology in a pragmatic way. It discusses ways and means of the applications of psychological rules, principles, theories, and techniques with reference to the real practical life situations.

Branches of Pure Psychology

General psychology: It deals with the general principles of psychology. General psychology describes the universal characteristics of human behavior and is concerned with the mental life of the normal human beings.

Abnormal psychology: It describes and explains the behavior of abnormal people in relation to their own environment. The etiological, symptoms and sign, syndromes, diagnosis, treatment, and rehabilitative aspects of the abnormalities of behavior from the subject matter of this branch.

Comparative and animal psychology: It studies the behavior of animals and compares and contrasts it with that of human beings.

Physiological psychology: Concerns the structure and functions of sense organs, nervous system muscles and glands underlying all behavior. It lays emphasis on the influence of bodily factors on human behavior.

Social psychology: This branch of psychology deals with the group behavior and inter-relationships of people with others, group dynamics, likes and dislikes interests and attitudes, social distance and prejudices of the people in their personal and social relationships from the subject matter of this branch.

Experimental psychology: It describes and explains the ways and means of carrying out psychological experiments following scientific methods in controlled or laboratory settings for the study of mental processes and behavior. This investigates the areas such as sensation, perception, learning, memory, motivation, forgetting, etc. in humans and other animals. This emphasis on basic research, i.e. knowledge for its own sake without much consideration as to its applications.

Genetic psychology/Developmental psychology: It studies the behavior from birth to old age, and the factors that influence the growth and development of human behavior. Special areas of interest include the development of language, social attachments, emotions, thinking and perception.

Clinical psychology: It focuses on understanding, diagnosing, and treating abnormal or deviant behaviors.

Para psychology: It deals with extra sensory perceptions, cases of re-birth-telepathy and allied problems.

Geo psychology: It describes and explains the relation of physical environment especially weather, climate, soil, and land scape with behavior.

Branches of Applied Psychology

Educational psychology: It is concerned with human learning and development in educational settings. It involves scientific study of techniques that can be used to enhance learning. It studies the teaching process, learner-learning process and the environment.

Industrial psychology: It tries to seek application of the psychological principles, theories and techniques for the study of human behavior in relation to industrial environment. It studies the taste and interests of the consumers, advertising and sale of products, selection, training and placing, solving labor problems, establishing harmonious relationship between employee and employer, strengthening morals of the workers and increasing production.

Legal psychology: This branch emphasis on the behavior of the persons like clients, criminals, witnesses, etc. in their own surroundings with the application of the psychological principles.

Community psychology: It studies the principles, ideals and points to view and help solve social problems and to help individuals adapt to their work and living groups.

Military psychology: It is concerned with the use of psychological principles and techniques in the world of military science. How to keep the morale of the soldiers and citizens high during war, how to fight war of propaganda and intelligence services, how to secure better recruitment and improvement strategies, organizational climate and leadership, etc.

Political psychology This branch of psychology deals itself with the use of psychological principles and techniques in studying the politics and deriving political gains. The knowledge of the dynamics of the group behavior, judgment of the public opinion, qualities of the leadership, psychology of the propaganda, suggestions and the art of diplomacy, etc.

PSYCHOLOGY AND NURSING

Why we need psychology in nursing sciences? The nursing profession deals with human behavior. Understanding and analyzing the different complex human interactions enable the nurse to serve the humanity in a better way. Primarily it helps

To know and understand herself: Psychology helps to know the individual himself or herself. Understanding motives, desires, emotions and ambitions of her helps to serve better. Individual nurse will realize how her personality is highly unique and complex, her thinking, feeling, reasoning, problem solving, decision making will help to understand the basic mental processes which lie behind behavior psychology will help to better assess her own abilities, limitations and her reaction to others and to various situations. This insights her to know her own behavior.

Psychology will help to understand others: Nurse has to serve, study and live with different categories of people in society. With scientific psychological background, the nurse will understand the people in a better way. She will study and learn why others differ in thinking, reasoning, likes and dislikes, abilities, beliefs and cultural customs. She will make allowances for other's short-comings and idiosyncrasies and will develop the positive attitude towards life and humanity. However, psychology will not solve all the problems of nurses but it enhances in understanding the human nature.

Study of the psychology will help: The nurse to appreciate the necessity of changing the environment or surrounding and guide her how to do this. The change in the environment is sometimes necessary for better adjustment and optimal living. For example, Wearing hearing aids will help to overcome the sensory deficiencies and to assist them in their attempts to achieve a more harmonious relationship with the surroundings.

Psychology will throw light on the interdependence: It includes the body, mind, and spirit. Knowing and applying the principles of psychology in work place helps to break the boredom and burnout. Coordial and harmony between herself and others at work and home will ease her anxiety and contributes for happy living.

In all these situations, psychology will make the nurse to stand in good stead, knowing herself better and insight's into other's behavior.

Methods of Psychology

The discovery of new knowledge in psychology is based on research tools and procedures. These procedures are known as methods of psychology. These are:

1. Experimental method
2. Correlational method
3. Observation method
4. Survey method
5. Clinical case method
6. Case studies
7. Testing.

Experimental Method

The scientific experiment is one of the powerful research tools to find out answers. The essential purpose is to discover what leads to what. In this method, strictly following the research steps to solve the problem and permitting for cause and effect relationships.

True/Classical Experiment

In psychological experiment, the researcher manipulates the some variables to observe the consequences. A variable is any changeable element or event that can be manipulated or studied in controllable or noncontrollable situations. The researcher tries to keep other conditions constant and looks forward for an effect or variation on the system under observation. Psychology is concerned with science of behavior; the psychologist looks for an effect of the experimental changes on behavior.

Variables

A variable that initiates some activity is known as a stimulus. The resulting activity or consequent event, if it involves action by any organism is called a response. The stimulus of wheezing in a bedridden person probably would awaken, which is a response. In research, stimuli are also known as S-variables and responses as R-variables.

Aspects of the organism are known as our variables. If the person were drugged, these conditions would influence her response to the shaking. A person's age, weight, gender, educational level and personality traits are difficult to define, but they influence the individual's response, which are in interest.

While conducting an experiment the investigator must generate hypothesis, subject selection, operationalizing the terms, finding out reliability and validity, control, analysis of results will be done in a scientific manner with advanced application of mathematical and statistical instruments.

Rule of one variable

In doing experiment, the investigator must decide which stimulus is variable to manipulate in relation to which response. The true or classical experimental method follows the rule of one variable, only one variable or multi is manipulated at any given moment. If an effect is observed, i.e. if change is observed in some response, then it is assumed to be the result of the manipulated factor, especially if other potentially influential factors are well controlled.

Independent variables (IV):

The investigator determines which variable is to be manipulated, that variable is known as independent variables. Changes in this factor are independent of all other aspects of the experiment. The researcher manipulates the IV in accordance with the basic problem in the study. If the investigator wants to know the influence of high temperature and pulse, temperature is considered as an independent variable.

Dependent Variable (DV)

The value of DV depends on the value of IV, the one independently chosen and directly manipulated by the experimenter.

Limitations

- Experiment method is not an ideal of choice if experiment might be dangerous for the subjects.
- The conclusions derived from experiment may be limited.
- Experimental method sometimes interferes with the very thing it is trying to measure.

Correlation method: This is a nonexperimental research design. A correlation is defined as a relationship between two variables such that when one variable systematically increases the other will systematically alter.

For example: There is a strong correlation between IQ and health. The more IQ one tends to be having very low/fewer health problems and the lower IQ level shows high health problems. Both the data are correlational and but can be find out the underlying cause and effect.

Observational method: The aim of the observational method is to study behavior in its natural setting, without asking any question or administrating any tests. The researcher simply observes and records what happens in the natural environment. He gathers ideas and makes hypotheses for subsequent testing in a more controlled setting.

Naturalistic observation is most often used to investigate behavior in the natural environment outside of the laboratory. Technically, a natural environment is defined as any environment that the researcher has not purposely manipulated for reasons of conducting study, i.e. one in which things are going on much as they would be regardless of the presence of the researcher, e.g. observing the children at playground.

Types of Natural Observation

The main aim of naturalistic observation is careful observing without any bias, e.g. a researcher might ask what behavior, if any, characterize the dreaming process? This question might be answered by careful observation by examining people who fall asleep. The types are:

Overt Observation

Here, the subject is aware of the observer, who may use checklists, rating scales and other devices for keeping systematic records of the behavior.

For example: observation of a sleeping person. In Overt observation, observer observes several gross body movements, changes in posture, relaxation movements, etc. After sometime, brief twitching movements of arms and legs, similar twitching in the face and heaving breathing.

Covert Observation

In covert observation, subjects are unaware that research data are being collected from them. The researcher proceeds in an unobstructive manner, insofar as possible. Observational method is greatly used in studying the behavior of animals and children. Thorndike has observed animals such as cats and white mice in mazes and puzzle boxes have given the idea of learning process.

For accurate results, one observation must be objective in nature. It must be free from biases and prejudices.

Limitations

- Does not yield in depth knowledge of any phenomena because nature is a complex phenomenon.
- Many number of factors influences cause and effect relations
- Risk of contamination in overt observation, while in covert observation, lacks the close contact with the subjects.
- Difficult to generalize the findings.

Survey method: A survey method is also one type of research method. A survey obtains information about the prevalence, distribution and inter-relation of variables within a population.

Surveys obtain information about people actions, knowledge, intentions, opinions and attitudes by means of self-report, i.e. study samples may respond to a set of questions. Surveys which yield quantitative data primarily may be cross-sectional or longitudinal (e.g. panel studies). Any information that can reliably be obtained by direct questioning can be gathered in a survey, but mostly includes brief responses (e.g. yes/no, always/sometimes/ never average/ good/excellent).

Survey data can be collected in a number of ways. Most popular method of collecting data is through interview. Interview may be personal and telephonic.

Case Studies

Case studies are in depth investigations of a single subject or a small number of entities. The entity may be an individual, of institution, community or other social unit. In a case study, researcher obtain descriptive information in detail and may examine relationships among different phenomena or trends over time. It attempts to analyze and understand issues that are important to the history, development or circumstances of the entity under study.

The main focus of case study is on determining the dynamics of why an individual thinks, behavior or develops in a particular manner rather than on what his or her status, progress or actions are studied over a considerable period. Data are collected prospectively as well as retrospective. It is a useful way to explore the phenomena in depth. The information obtained can be used to develop hypotheses and can further be tested. The intensive probing that characterizes case studies often leads to insights about previously unsuspected relationships. It also helps to clarify the concepts regarding phenomena. For example, psychotherapy.

Drawbacks:

- Difficult to impart objectivity
- Lacks generalizability.

Testing

Test can be used to investigate the behavior. These can be valuable research instrument. Tests are used to measure many aptitudes, abilities and personalities. Test also may make it possible to measure various characteristics of people by testing large groups of individuals at one time. So these are used in education, business, clinicals, the military, and industry. These may be administered individually, often for the purpose of clinical, intellectual or personality assessment.

For examples: IQ test—to test intelligence.
Rorschach ink blots test to—test personality.
Minnesota multiphasic personality inventory (MMPT)—to test personality type.
Thematic appreciation test (TAT).

SUMMARY POINTS

- Psychology is the study of behavior and mental processes.
- There are many different areas of specialization within psychology. Among them are neuropsychological, psychobiological, developmental, general, educational, legal, military, industrial, para psychology and clinical psychology.
- Psychology was born of two parents, philosophy and physiology. The union of the philosopher's questions and the psychologist's careful scientific investigations and analysis lead to psychological research which began in a laboratory in Leipzig, Germany in 1879.
- The first experimental physiology laboratory was started by Wilhelm Wundt who was interested in analyzing the mind. This has given birth to Structuralism, relied on the technique of introspection.
- John Dewey and William James introduced functionalism. They believed that human consciousness and behavior must serve a function.

- John B Watson developed an objective system of psychology he called behaviorism. The product of this, S-R psychology that values our behavior is determined by our immediate environment or previous history of learning.
- In Germany, Structuralism was born. Gestalt psychologist argue that conscious sensations can be examined but that the whole experience must be taken for what it is.
- Psychoanalytical theory was developed by a Viennese physician, Sigmund Freud. Its roots are in neurology and medicine.
- Humanistic psychology differs from other philosophies. Humanists believe that people have free will and a need to achieve self-actualization.
- The biological approach to study of psychology is the new trend. It concerns itself with the investigation of the brain, nervous system, genetic inheritance and biology of the organism as pertain to behavior and mental processes.
- Cognitive psychology is the study of internal mental processes, which include thinking, memory, concept formation, forgetting and the processing of information.
- All scientific research relies on systematic and objective methods of observing, recording and describing events. The experimental study is one of the most powerful tools to conduct the study.
- Data from correlations are valuable because they allow us to make predictions. However, cause-effect relationships cannot make merely because a correlation exists.
- In naturalistic observation, researcher refrains from directly interacting with the subjects they are observing. Naturalistic observation is most often used to investigate behavior in natural environment in which the researcher refrains from manipulation.
- Other research tools used by psychological researchers include case studies, surveys, clinical case methods and testing.
- All the work in scientific psychology is aimed at a common goal to predict, to explain and eventually to control behavior.

Questions for Introspection

1. Define psychology. Describe its meaning.
2. What are the various branches of psychology?
3. Why psychology is considered as a science?
4. Why nurses have to study psychology?
5. What are the different research approaches in psychology?
6. Explain the term behavior by providing an illustration.

Chapter 2

Biological Basis of Psychology

MIND – BODY RELATIONSHIP

Mind

One of the iconic questions in psychology is mind. What is mind? Where it is? And how it is? The definition of psychology depicts as a science of human behavior which expresses the mental processes and experiences. To explain the mind is a great task. Confusion and complexity prevails about mind. Earlier, according to Vedanta, the philosophers and rhishis, named it as 'Chitta' which means mind. The theorists who assume the mind and body are separate entities, describe mind as something intangible, differs from body/matter/or soma; which is concrete and tangible, But this not a suitable explanation. It has been proved that mind and body are not separate entities, but they are interrelated and inter-connected. Therefore, mind is a function of body; it does not exist in apart.

Mind is the sum total of various mental processes such as thinking, imagining, reasoning, and feeling, remembering and judging. It is not a separate object which possesses the mental activities. Mind is conglomeration of thoughts. The newer perspective that mind is nothing but thinking. Thinking itself is Mind.

Mind grows as we grow from infancy to adulthood. It becomes more complex with advance years, i.e. our psychological processes become richer and more complex day by day as we grow, e.g. we can observe a difference between thinking and reasoning of an adult and a child of five years.

Aspects of Conscious, Preconscious/Subconscious and Unconsciousness

The forefathers of newer theorists in psychology thought that mind was nothing but 'conscious'. So, earlier days, psychology was defined as study of consciousness. It was regarded as the sum total of all conscious mental processes only mental processes which are aware at a time. The modern scientists believe that mind is more than consciousness. They thought that it includes preconscious and unconscious process all these three constitute our mind. We can conclude that mind is one having three levels of consciousness. Primarily, the individual is aware about his mental process, i.e. the 'conscious'. The other one whether is not aware fully of our mental processes is called 'unconsciousness'. The third level, we are not conscious of our mental processes at a certain level of time but we are aware of them before and can again be aware after some time, if we try, this is preconscious/ subconsciousness.

Consciousness

The conscious process of the mind is known as consciousness. *For example*: Sitting in a lecturer hall. You know what is going on in a classroom, who is lecturing? What, etc. Thus, observing, attending to something, reasoning, thinking, imagining are the functions of consciousness mental processes.

When we are conscious, we monitor the internal and external environment, but also we seek to control ourselves and our environment. In short consciousness involves (a) monitoring ourselves and our environment, so that percepts, memories and thoughts are represented in awareness and (b) controlling ourselves and our environment, so that we are able to initiate and terminate behavioral and cognitive activities.

Preconsciousness/subconsciousness/fore-consciousness processes are those of which you were aware before and which can be recollected with effort. At this moment they are just below the margin of consciousness. The difference between conscious processes and preconscious processes is that the latter the attribute of consciousness is temporarily missing; e.g. when we are deeply absorbed in studies, the hungriness /clock goes on unnoticed.

Memories that are accessible to consciousness are called preconscious memories. They include specific memories of personal events, as well as the information accumulated over a life time, such as one's knowledge of the meaning of words, the layout of the city or the location of a particular building. They also include knowledge about learned skills like the procedures involved in driving car or the sequence of steps in administering IV injection. These procedures, once mastered, generally operate outside conscious awareness, but when our attention is called to them we are capable of describing the steps in detail.

The unconscious processes constitute the unconsciousness. This is the processes of which we are totally unaware and which are incapable of becoming conscious unless special methods are used, e.g. psychoanalytic procedure. These processes lie buried deep down in the hidden recesses of the mind very much below the level of consciousness. It was Freud and his followers strongly advocated that some emotionally painful memories and wishes are repressed, i.e. diverted to the unconsciousness where they may continue to influence our actions even though we are not aware of them. Thoughts and impulses repressed to the unconscious, where they may continue to influence our actions even though we are not aware of them. Thoughts and impulses repressed to the unconscious cannot enter our consciousness; but they can affect us in indirect or disguised ways—through dreams, irrational behaviors, mannerisms and slips of tongue. The term "Freudian Slip" is commonly used to refer to unintentional remarks that are assumed to reveal hidden impulses.

For example: I am sad you are better, when intending to say "I" am glad you are better.

It is to be noted that there are no compartments in our mind to store preconscious or unconscious processes separately. Pre and unconsciousness are a part of same mind that the conscious processes belong to. The former are simply those mental processes which we forgotten, either temporarily or less in a permanent way. Their connections of our conscious processes are broken for the time being.

Analysis of Psychological Phenomena

Any conscious experience consists of three distinct psychological processes. These are thinking, knowing, feeling and striving, *for example*: when you are listening to a lecture on a nursing procedure, you understand the meaning of words which includes thinking, thus know certain facts, and are learning them. You also 'feeling' pleased/displeased with the class and is enjoying or bored by it. Lastly, you may 'wish' that the class may be continued or discontinued.

These three processes of thinking/knowing, feeling and willing are called cognition, affect, and conation. These three modes are known as being conscious. Every conscious experience is thinking, knowing something, is pleasant or unpleasant and is striving towards something.

One more factor we should keep in mind that our conscious experiences are never purely cognitive or affective or conative. Every mental experience is a complex whole having elements of thinking, knowing, feeling or wishing and striving. These elements are present in all our conscious experiences, in a greater or less degree.

A cognitive process or a thinking experience is not devoid of feeling or conation, but the more part is cognition in it. An affective process is not devoid of cognition/conation itself, it has more feeling element in it. Similarly, a conative processes has more of doing element in it, and although it is not devoid of the elements of cognition and affect. A process is called cognitive, affective or conative depending on the element that predominates in it.

To achieve a good health, all these three elements have to operate in a harmonious way. Any one element or all elements operate in a disfashioned or disorganized way leads to psychological problems.

Mind-body Relationship

Our behavior involves both body and mind. Both will interact with one another. Mental functions and physical states affect each other. This is the modern concept called "interactionism". The old concept of parallelism was mind and body ran in parallel grooves without interacting on each other.

The human nervous and endocrine glands are responsible for our thinking, feeling and wishing. The following examples highlight how bodily functions affects mental functioning in a normal healthy person:

- Increase in blood pressure leads to psychological over activity.
- Fatigue of the body induces, decreased concentration and sense of proportion.

- Constipation can cause irritability and depression.
- Excessive thyroid secretion leads to mental restlessness and anxiety where as under secretion of thyroid glands leads to lethargy of mind and body. The mind, too affects our bodily functions.
  a. Mind motivates all physical and motor activities.
  b. Emotions and strong feelings affect the body inside and outwardly. Unpleasant emotions causes psychosomatic symptoms. Emotional conflicts are responsible for various neurotic disorders such as gastrointestinal problems like peptic ulcers, ulcerative colitis, etc.
  c. Excessive thinking and concentration can cause physical fatigue.

The mind or psychological processes are always connected to a body, but very intimately connected with brain, for example:

- The more intelligent animals have better developed brains. Human beings are the super thinkers than any animal.
- If any injury/disease occur to the brain, it affects the mental processes. Individuals affected with brain damage suffers from deficiency in thinking, reasoning and in other higher mental functions.
- . The nerves carry the impulse of bodily changes to brain and then alone do mental processes take place. When we experience any pain or pin prickle in leg, our nerves carry the message to the brain and the mental experience of pain is felt.

Now, it is understood that diseases/disorders are not only related to bodily functions for but it also includes psychic/mind functions. The newer disease in medicine is believed that many somatic or bodily complaints are caused and accentuated by psychic and mental factors. Hence, the management is diverted toward both sources of illness the emotions and the bodily causes.

Behavioral Genetics

Genetics and Behavior: Heredity and Environment

The word genetics was coined by Batson in 1906. It has been derived from the Greek word 'gene' which means 'to become'/ 'to grow into'. Therefore, genetics is the science of coming into being.

"Genetics" is that branch of biological sciences which deals with the transmission of characteristics from parents to offspring. Medical genetics focuses on the inheritance of the population.

It is also defined as the science that deals with the study of heredity (inheritance of traits from one generation to another) and variations (differences among the individual's of same parents or a species) is known as genetics.

Gene: Structure and Characteristics

A gene is the basic physical and functional unit of heredity. This is made up of DNA, act as RNA instructor to make molecules called proteins. In human beings, genes vary in size from a few hundred DNA bases to more than two million bases. The Human Genome Project has estimated that humans have between 20,000 to 25,000 genes. Every individual has two copies of each gene, one inherited from each parent. Most genes are the same in all people, but a small number of genes (less than 1% of the total) are slightly different between people. Alleles are forms of the same gene with small differences in their sequence of DNA bases. These small differences contribute to each person's unique physical and psychological features.

Structure of the Gene

Chemical Structure

The genetic information of all living organism, except the RNA viruses, is stored in DNA. DNA and RNA are collectively called nucleic acids. In 1869, F Meisher isolated substances from cell nuclei and named it as "nuclein." Due to their acidic nature, they were named as nucleic acids.

Nucleic acids are macromolecules composed of repeating subunits called nucleotides. Each nucleotide is composed of (1) a phosphate group (2) a five carbon sugar (or pentose) and 3) a cyclic nitrogen containing compound called a base.

Diagram

(1) A phosphate group

O^-
$O^- - P = O$
O^-

(2) A five carbon sugar or pentose

(a) mRMA

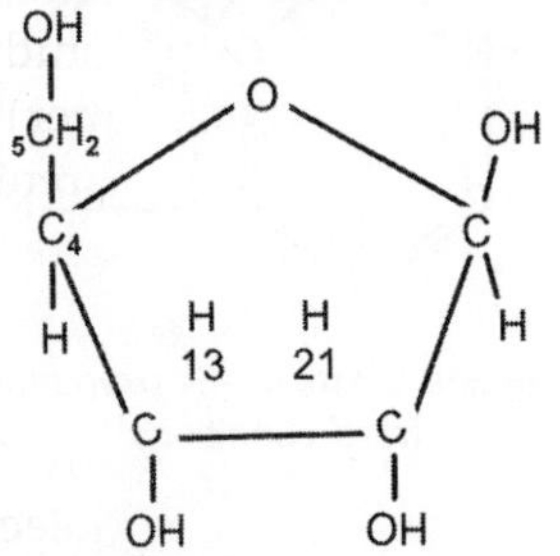

IN DNA

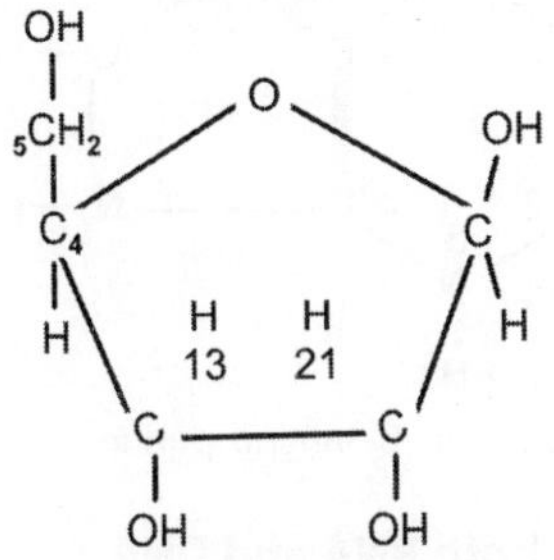

In DNA, the sugar is 2- deoxyribose, in RNA the sugar is ribose. There are four different nitrogen bases commonly found in DNA: adenine, guanine, thymine, and cytosine. RNA also usually contains adenine, guanine, and cytosine but has a different base Uracil, in place of thymine. Adenine and guanine are double ring bases called purines: cytosine, thymine and uracil are single ring bases called pyrimidines. So, both DNA and RNA consist of four nucleotides, two purine nucleotides and two pyrimidine nucleotides. RNA usually exists as a single stranded molecule that is composed of a long sequence of nucleotides. DNA is mostly double stranded.

3. A cyclic nitrogen containing base.

(A) In RNA only (rare condition)

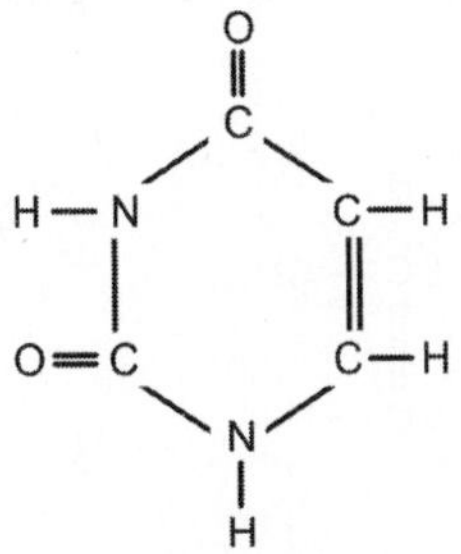

Uracil (2,4 - oxypyrimidine)

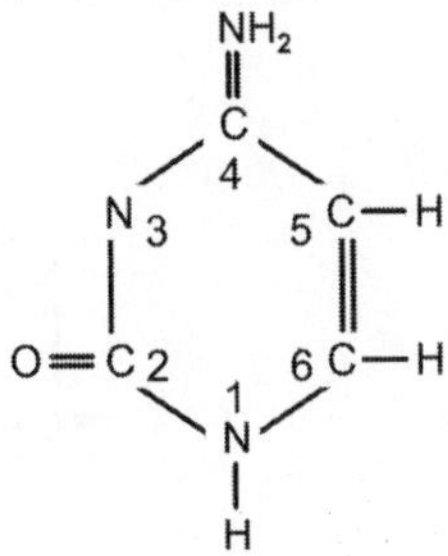

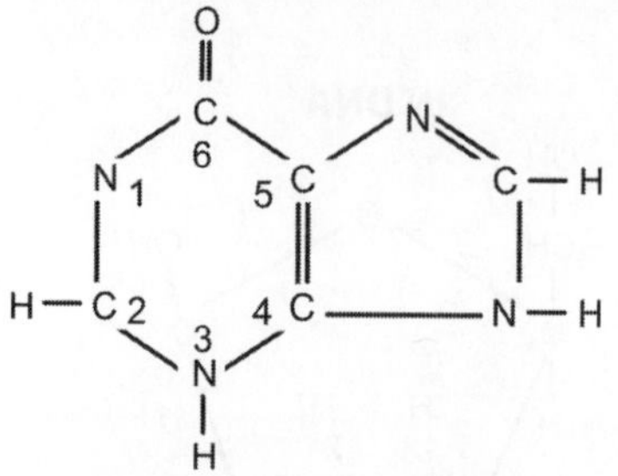

Adenine -6- amino purine

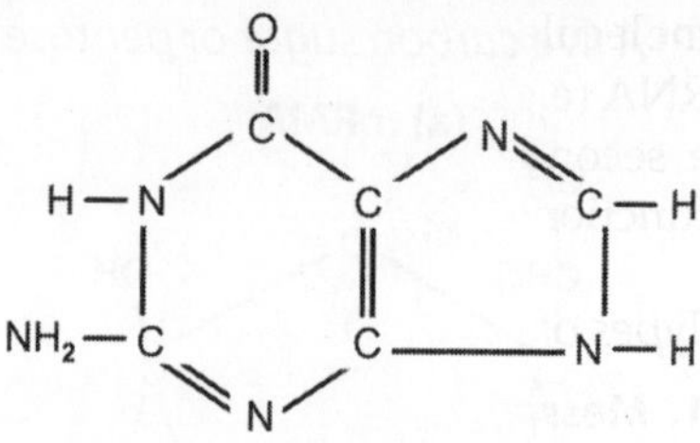

Guaine 2 amino -6- oxypurine
(rare conditions)

(B) In both RNA and DNA

(C) Cytosine (4 amino-2- oxypyrimidine)

(D) In DNA only

DNA is a nucleic acid that contains instructions for the development and function of living things. The main role of DNA in the cell is the long term storage of information. In animal, DNA is stored inside the cell nucleus, while in bacteria the DNA is in the cell's cytoplasm. DNA does not act directly on other molecules, rather, various enzymes act on DNA and copy its information into either more DNA, in DNA replication or transcribe in into protein. In chromosomes, chromatin proteins such as histones compact and organize DNA, as well as helping control its interactions with other proteins in the nucleus.

Ribonucleic Acid (RNA)

RNA is usually single stranded virus. RNA contains ribose sugar and pyrimidines cytosine and uracil. However, purines in both RNA and DNA are the same adenine and guanine. RNA

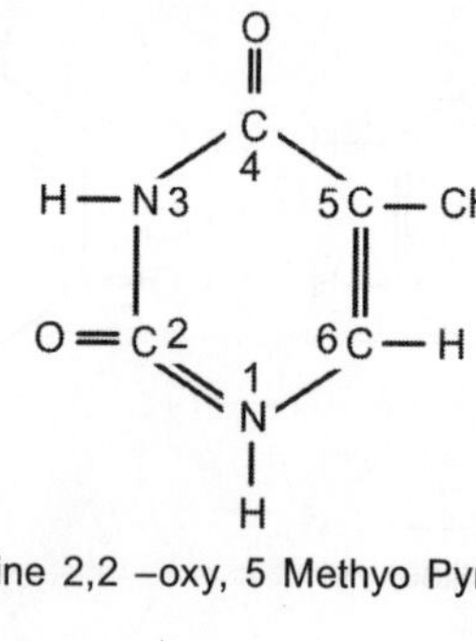

Thymine 2,2 –oxy, 5 Methyo Pyrimidine

molecules are much shorter than DNA molecules. Several types f RNA (e.g. t RNA and, RNA) contain double stranded regions and a secondary structure which helps RNA's to perform different functions.

Types of RNA: Human cell contains 4 types of RNA.

1. Messenger RNA (mRNA): It carries genetic information from the DNA in the nucleus to the cytoplasm for the synthesis of the polypeptide.

2. Ribosomal RNA (rRNA): It is the constituent of ribosomes. It is 4 types 18s, 5s, 5.8s and 28s. It performs various functions including the formation of peptide bond between amino acids during protein synthesis when the ribosome moves along the mRNA.

3. Transfer RNA (tRNA): tRNA molecules bind to specific amino acids and bring them to the site of protein synthesis on the ribosome, where they read the coded message in the mRNA and fit the amino acids accordingly in the polypeptide chain being synthesized. There are at least 31 types of tRNA for 20 types of amino acids.

4. Small nuclear RNA (Sn RNA's): These are the constituents of splicrosomes, which remove the noncoding regions (introns) from the primary transcripts (hnRNAs) of genes and splice the coding regions (exons) together to construct the functional mRNA molecules. It is noted that most eukaryotic genes are split genes containing noncoding regions or introns and coding regions or exons.

Other types of RNA's:

1. Genetic RNA: In RNA viruses, the genetic information is stored in the RNA molecules, e.g. most of the plant viruses. RNA may be single stranded (Polio virus) or double stranded (e.g. Reo virus).

2. Nongenetic RNAs: They may perform various functions in the cells. These include:

a. Antisense RNA, called micRNA (messenger RNA inhibiting complementary RNA) is complementary to mRNA and is used for gene regulation.
b. ScRNA (small cytoplasmic RNA) is associated with proteins sc RNP's or scyrps.

c. Guide RNA (RNA) cosynthesized from minicircle mitochondrial DNA (mt, DNA) is used for RNA editing leading to modification of transcribed RNA. Thus, it has a catalytic for such catalytic RNA's are called ribozymes.
d. Small nucleolar RNA (sno RNA). It is found in nucleolus and is involved in processing of ribosomal RNA.
e. The replication of DNA and transcription are the main functions of the gene.

Gene Mutation and Health

For normal functioning, each cell depends on thousands of proteins to do their job in the right places at right time. Sometimes, gene mutations prevent one or more of these proteins from working properly. By changing a gene's instructions for making a protein a mutation can cause the protein to malfunction or to be missing entirely. When a mutation alters a protein that plays a critical role in the body, it can disrupt normal growth and development or cause medico-psychological condition. A condition caused by mutations in one or more genes is called a genetic disorder.

Gene mutations are so severe that they prevent an embryo from surviving until birth. These changes occur in genes that are essential for development, and often disrupt the development of an embryo in its earliest stages. Because these mutations have very serious effects, they are incompatible with life. It is important to know that genes themselves do not cause disease, genetic disorders are caused by mutations that make gene function improperly.

For example: the cystic fibrosis gene-causes cysticfibrosis. All people, including those with out cystic fibrosis have a version of the CFTR gene.

Mechanism of Inheritance

The disorders can be said as "running in a family; shows more than one person has the condition in a family. Disorders that affect multiple family members are caused by gene mutations which can be inherited (parent to child) other conditions that appear to run in fit are not inherited. Instead environmental factors such as diet economical condition or a combination of genetic and environmental factors are responsible for disorders.

Gregor Mandel's Law of Inheritance

The genes provide all information to growth and development. When a gene is changed different message is passed to the cells. It makes the genes faulty is called mutation. A faulty (mutated) gene may cause a problem in the development and functioning of body. Our genes are inherited by our forefathers. The great majority of genes come in pairs, the exceptions being the genes on the sex chromosomes (X and Y) of a male. The Mendelian inheritance applies when a characteristic or set of characteristics is due to the information contained in a single gene pair. The characteristic may be "usual" or "it may not", it could be a genetic condition. The inheritance depends on whether the faulty gene is part of one of the external chromosome called an autosome, or on the X-chromosome which is one of the sex chromosomes. It depends on whether the mutation that makes the gene faulty is "recessive" or "dominant".

PATTERNS OF INHERITANCE

Some genetic disorders are caused by mutations in a single gene. These conditions are usually inherited in one of several straightforward patterns, depending on the gene involved.

Autosomal Dominant

One mutated copy of the gene in each cell is sufficient for a person to be affected by an autosomal dominant disorder. Each affected person usually has one affected parent. Autosomal dominant disorders tend to occur in every generation of an affected family.

For example: Hunting ton's disease - Breast cancer
Marfan syndrome - Neurofibromatosis type -I
Colon cancer.

Autosomal Recessive

Two mutated copies of the gene are present in each cell when a person has an autosomal recessive disorder. An affected person usually has unaffected parents who each carry a single copy of the mutated gene (called as carriers). Autosomal recessive disorders are typically not seen in every generation of an affected family.

For example: Cystic fibrosis
Thalassemia
Sickle cell anemia
Phyenelkentonuria.

Sex-linked Inheritance

a. X-Linked Dominant Inheritance

This is caused by mutations in genes on the X-chromosome. Families with this disorder often have both affected males and females in each generation. A striking characteristic of X-linked inheritance is that fathers cannot pass x-linked traits to their sons. *For example*: Fragile X-syndrome.

b. X-Linked Recessive

These are caused by mutations in the genes on the X-chromosome. Males are more frequently affected than females, and the chance of passing on the disorder differs between man and women. The affected families often have affected males, but rarely affected females, in each generation.

For example: Hemophilia
Hunting syndrome
Duchenne muscular dystrophy

c. X-linked Recessive (affected fathers):

Here it affected father.

d. X-linked Recessivè

In this inheritance, mother is the carrier.

Codominant Pattern of Inheritance

In codominant inheritance, two different versions (alleles) of a gene can be expressed, and each version makes a slightly different protein. Both alleles influence the genetic trait or determine the characteristic's of the genetic condition.

For example: ABO blood group.
Alpha-1 antitrypsin deficiency.

Mitochondrial Pattern of Inheritance

This is also known as maternal inheritance, applies to gene in mitochondrial DNA. Mitochondria, with are structures in each cell that convert molecules into energy, each contain a small amount of DNA. Because only egg cells contribute mitochondria to the developing embryo, only females can pass on mitochondrial conditions to their children. These can appear in every generation of a family and can affect both males and females, but fathers do not pass mitochondrial traits to their children.
For example: Leber's hereditary optic neuropathy (LHON).

Multifactorial Pattern of Inheritance

Multifactorial inheritance conditions are believed to be the result of multiple mutations and environmental influence that combine to cause birth defects/disorders. Genetic conditions with a multifactorial cause trend to cluster in families but do not follow the characteristic pattern of inheritance with single gene disorder.

For example: Congenital heart disease
Cleft lip/ palate
Neural tube defect.

For harmonious psychological development, the genetic make-up must be in normal ways. Any alteration in genetic make-up inheritance alters the psychological development in forecoming development.

BRAIN AND BEHAVIOR

Behavior, from blinking an eye to playing football to designing a web program, depends on the integration of many different processes within the body. This integration is provided by the nervous system with the help of endocrine system. For example, Consider, you have to stop your car at red signal. First you must see the red light: this means that the light must register on one set of your eyes. Neural impulses from eyes are relayed to your brain where the stimulus is analyzed and compared with information about past events stored in memory and to recognize that a red light means 'stop'. The process of moving foot to the brake and pressing initiated by the motor areas of the brain that control the muscles of your leg and foot. In order to send the proper signals of these muscles, the brain must know where your foot is as well as where you want it to go. The brain maintains a register of the position of body parts relative to one another, uses to plan directed movements. You do not stop the car with one sudden movement of your leg. A specialized part of the brain receives continuous feedback from leg and foot muscles so that you are aware of how much pressure is being exerted and can alter your movements accordingly. At the same time, eyes and some other body parts senses tell you how quickly the car is stopping. If the light turned red as you were speeding toward the intersection some of your endocrine glands would also be activated, leading to enhanced heart rate, rapid respiration and other metabolic changes associated with fear, these processes speed your reactions in an emergency. The whole activities of this process is transmitted by large network of nerve cells or neurons.

Our nervous system, sense organs, muscles and glands enable us to be aware of and to adjust to our environment. Our perception of events depends on how our sense organs detect stimuli and how our brain interprets information arising from the senses. Much of our behavior is motivated by such needs as hunger, thirst and the avoidance of fatigue or pain. Our ability to use language, to think and to solve problems depends on a brain that is incredibly complex. However, the specific patterns of electrical and chemical events in the brain are the very basis of our most intricate thought/ideas.

Nervous System

The nervous system is a complex system. At birth, it is not perfectly suited for adulthood. It gradually grows and develops. As it grows, gradual differentiation of function and response among various parts of body is seen.

For example: a child has to move his whole body to get a toy placed before him whereas adult takes it by stretching his arm.

Parts of the Nervous System

It consists of the brain, the spinal cord and the nerves which the brain and the spinal cord send off to all parts of the body. Generally, the nervous system is divided into three main parts:

a. The peripheral nervous system.
b. The central or cerebrospinal nervous system and
c. The automatic or sympathetic nervous system.

Peripheral Nervous System

The peripheral nervous system consists of two types of nerves which receive stimuli or transmit responses. The nerves which receive stimuli or impressions from external environment and carry them to the brain are called sensory or afferent nerves. On other side, there are nerves which originate from the brain a message or impulse for some particular action. These nerves are called motor or efferent nerves.

For example: putting leg on thorn. The afferent nerves will carry message that the sensation gives, namely injury to leg. The brain then takes stock of the happening, understands the situation and sends a message back along the efferent nerves to the leg muscles, informing them to move the leg. The whole process takes almost instantaneously and also simultaneously.

The structural unit of these nerves is a neuron or a nerve cell.

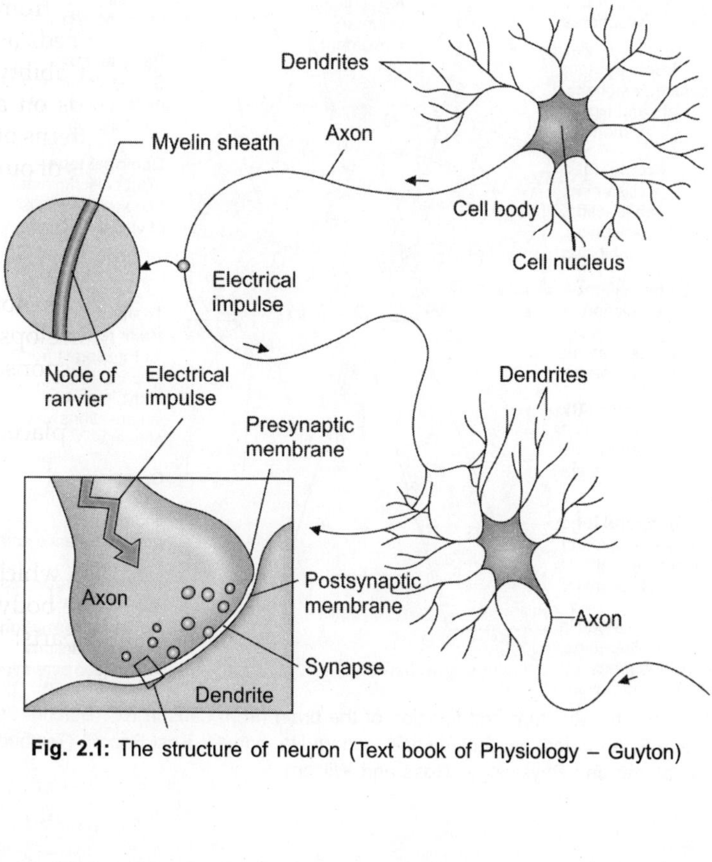

Fig. 2.1: The structure of neuron (Text book of Physiology – Guyton)

Every neuron consists of cell body, an axon, and dendrites. The information is carried from one neuron to another. The dendrites acts like receiving station that pick of impulses; the axons passes them to neurons through dendrites. These nerve fibers extend from the cell body in different directions. When two neurons lie very close to each other, impulses passes through one to one. The connection is known as synapse. These nerves acts like a communication system between the brain and various parts of the body. They merely carry messages to and from the brain, cannot feel any sensation or they cannot issue a command.

Central Nervous System

The central nervous system comprises the brain and the spinal cord.

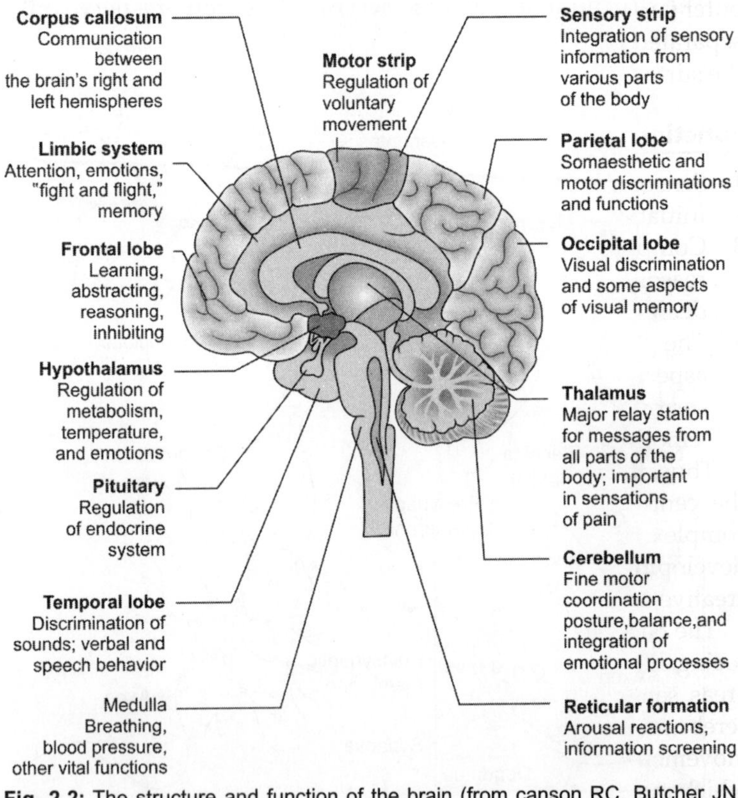

Fig. 2.2: The structure and function of the brain (from canson RC, Butcher JN, Mineka S: Abnormal psychology and modern life, edn 11, Bost Bacon) (Textbook of Anatomy and Physiology Ross and Wilson)

Brain

It lies within cranial cavity. It consists of following parts:

Forebrain : Cerebrum, thalamus
Midbrain : Midbrain
Hind brain : Pons
Medulla oblongata (Brain stem)
cerebellum.

Cerebrum

It is the largest part of the brain and occupies the most cranial cavity. It consists of right and left hemispheres which are connected by carpous collosum. Both hemispheres are separated by falx cerebri. The superficial part is composed of nerve cells of grey matter (cortex) and deeper matter is known as white matter. The outer surface of cerebral cortex shows many infoldings. These are separated by sulci or fissures. These convolutions greatly increase the surface area of the cerebrum. The elevations are called as gyri.

Functions of the Cerebrum

1. Sensory perception and temperature maintenance.
2. Initiation and control of voluntary muscle contractions.
3. Complex integrative functions as memory, emotions, thinking reasoning, judgment, personality traits and intelligence are dealt with by the cerebrum.
4. The limbic system with hypothalamus governs emotional aspects of behavior such as pain, pleasure, anger, rage, fear, sorrow, sexual feelings, and affection. It is also called as 'emotional' brain.

Thus, the cerebrum of the brain is the organ of consciousness, the centre for learning, the organ of integration for unifying complex responses and the organ which makes possible mental development, intelligent behavior and all kinds of adaptable and creative activities.

The back parts of the cerebrum constitute the sensory areas of seeing, hearing, tasting, smelling and touching or feeling. To these areas sensory nerves carry impressions. The front parts of the cerebrum have motor areas and are then concerned with volition, movement and effort. From these parts arise the motor nerves which move the different limbs and organs of the body.

Cerebellum (Little brain)

It lies beneath the back part of the cerebrum and weighs about one tenth of entire brain. It exercises an influence over the muscles of the body by regulating their movements. It unites and coordinates the movements and muscles and limbs of our body so that the functions can be coordinated, e.g. walking, running, jumping. Thus, the cerebellum is concerned with the coordination of the muscular movements and maintains the body equilibrium.

Thalamus

The thalamus measures about 3 cm in length. It consists of paired oval masses of grey matter organized into nuclei. It is concerned with the reception of sensory impulses from sub cortical level and spinal cord and relayed on to the sensory area of the cerebral cortex. It is postulated that, it contains centers of control for emotional behavior.

Medulla Oblongata

Medulla extends from the pons and it is continuous below with the spinal cord. It is about 2.5 cm long and has a pyramid shape. It is composed of white matter which passes between the brain and spinal cord and grey matter lies centrally. Nerve currents pass through it to the cerebellum and also down to the spinal cord. It is the seat of reflex connections and as such, controls the pupillary reflex, sneezing and winking. It governs the activity of vital organs such as heart, lungs and blood vessels and controls the bodily functions of respiration and circulation. If the upper portion of the medulla is injured, all the connections between the cerebrum and the rest of the body are broken, if the lower portion is injured, the respiratory and circulatory functions of lungs and heart will be affected.

Spinal Cord

The spinal cord is a part of the CNS situated in the vertebral column. It is almost cylindrical in shape, surrounded by meninges and cerebrospinal fluid. It is continuous as medulla oblongata till coccyx. The length of spinal cord is about 45 cm. It extends from the upper border of atlas to lower border of 1st lumber vertebra.

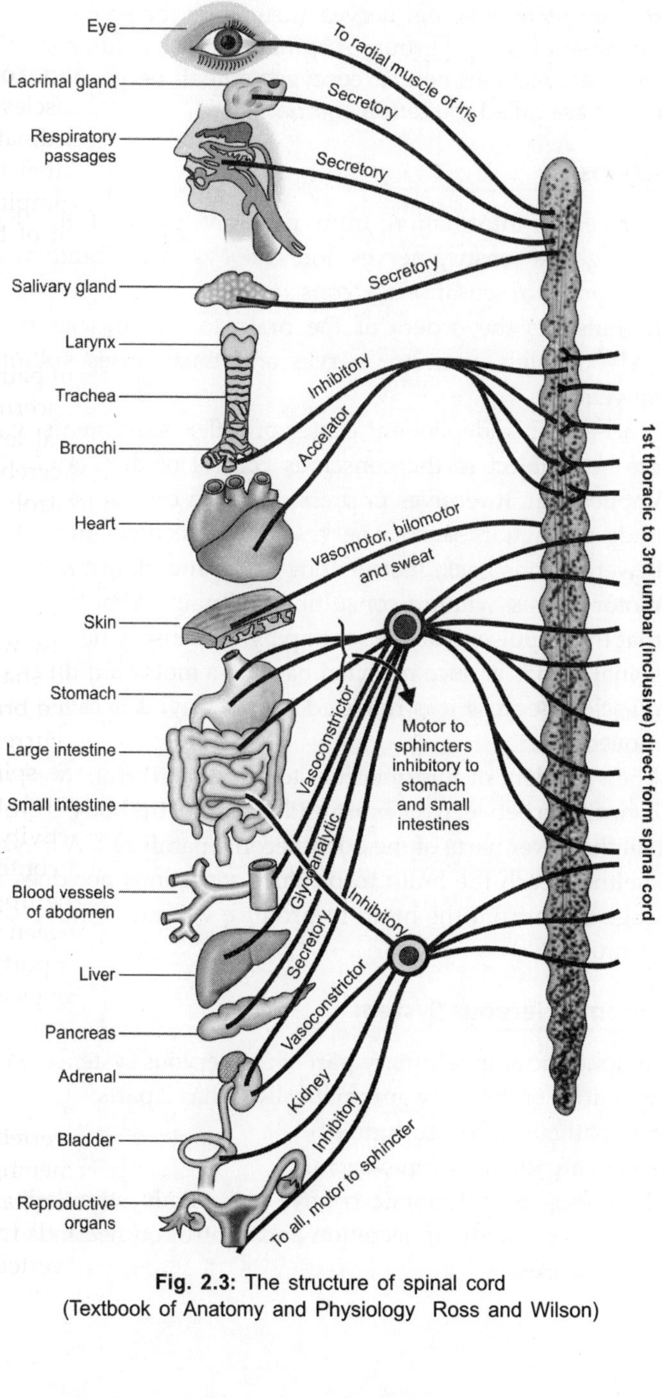

Fig. 2.3: The structure of spinal cord
(Textbook of Anatomy and Physiology Ross and Wilson)

Thirty one pairs of spinal nerves arise along the spinal cord. At the terminal of cord, a group of spinal nerves, i.e. lumbar spinal nerves, sacro-spinal nerve, coccygeo-spinal nerve and filum terminale are called the cauda equina.

Functions

1. It receives information from different parts of the body through its sensory nerves and conveys to the brain where they produce sensations of consciousness.
2. It transmits the orders of the brain to the muscles of the body through its motor nerves and thus causes voluntary movements.
3. It acts as an independent center of reflex movements which are not subject to the conscious control of the cortex. This implies that, it receives impressions from certain parts of the body through its sensory nerves, and on its own authority, as it were, sends back, instructions to the muscles, through the motor nerves, without consulting the brain. What happens is that the impulse which is sent up by the sensory nerves to the spinal cord is at once reflected back on a motor impulse to the muscles. Because it is reflected in this way, it is called reflex movement.

When accident or injury occurs to spinal cord from the brain, the connection between the brain and the rest of the body is broken and all the lower parts of the body become paralyzed. A message can neither reach the brain to produce sensations nor does any message come from the brain to produce voluntary movements in the muscles.

Autonomic Nervous System

The autonomic or involuntary part of the nervous system controls the functions of the body automatically. It has 2 parts:

1. Sympathetic (Thoraco-lumber)
2. Parasympathetic (Cranio-sacral).

The effects of autonomic control are mainly stimulation or depression of glandular secretion and control on heart rate and smooth muscles.

Sympathetic Nervous System

Sympathetic nervous system consists of 3 neurons conveying impulses from their origin in the hypothalamus reticular formation and medulla oblongata to effector organs and tissues.

Sympathetic Chain

A pair of sympathetic nerves situated on either side of vertebral column extending from the base of the skull to anterior surface of coccyx. In the chain, there are accumulations of nerve cells to form ganglia. There may be 22 to 24 sympathetic ganglia. The preganglonic fibers from the spinal cord relay in these ganglia. Then the postganglionic fibers come out from these chains to supply effector organs. The sweat glands, the skin and blood vessels of skeletal muscles are supplied by only sympathetic nerve fibers.

Parasympathetic Nervous System

It is connected to the brain and the lower part of spinal cord. It tends to be active when we are calm and relaxed. The messages conveyed by the nerve fibers of this system direct the organs to do just the opposite of what the sympathetic system had asked. In other words, it directs the body organs to return to a normal state after an emergency situation has over. As a result, breathing calms down, heart rate becomes normal, stomach muscles relax, the pupils of the eyes constrict and the blood pressure is lowered.

Nervous System and Behavior

Functions of the Brain

The brain is the seat of all functions of the body. According to Franz, and Lashley, they postulated two distinct laws on cerebral localizations, namely, the law of mass action and the law of equipotentiality. The law of mass action states that the learned process disintegrate in the ratio in which the cortex nerve fibers are destroyed, and the law of equipotentiality states that every point of cortex has equal potential. The potentiality of cortex destroys in the ratio the potentiality destroys.

Motor Area: This look likes narrow strips in front of the central fissure. These areas belonging to each hemisphere control the movements of the body of its opposite side by instructing the muscles and glands what to do next. While movements of the toes, feet and legs are controlled by the centers lying at the top of in motor region, the movements of the mouth and tongue are controlled by the centers located in the lower region. Movements of these parts of the body get paralyzed when accident occurs, the associated motor area suffers destruction.

Frontal Lobes

The functions of frontal lobes are not yet well understood. Damage to these areas has resulted in behavioral changes. These may be emotional dulling, distractibility and difficulty in executing sequence of behavior.

Bodily sensory area: This area is connected with sensation such as temperature, pain and feeling.

Visual area: Visual center is located in the occipital lobe, back of each hemisphere. Visual center helps in discriminating and identifying the object's size, shape, distance and color. Damage to this center can cause blindness.

Speech area: Speech area is responsible for the controlling the conduct of speech lies in frontal lobe. Speech hinderance and speech disorders will be seen if damage occurs to this center.

Auditory area: These are located at the side of each hemisphere in the temporal lobes. Their function is to provide various auditory experiences in terms of identification and discrimination of various sounds stimuli present in the environment.

Temporal lobes: This is responsible for maintenance of temperament.

Association area: This lies beneath the forehead. Their function is to influence sensory or motor responses but also concerned with higher intellectual functions like thinking, reasoning, and problem solving.

NERVOUS SYSTEM AND BEHAVIOR

Brain is the finest gift of God to mankind. It plays a significant role in our activities. To a great extent, behavior is controlled and co-coordinated by nervous system. The sense organs bear significance by nervous system. Normal development helps to grow and functions the nervous system in a healthy way. Physical, emotional, psychological and all round learning is influenced by nervous system. Autonomic nervous system controls the activities of involuntary processes like circulation of blood, respiration and action of glands. Our emotional states like happiness, anger/ violence also cause change in the secretion of hormones by glands. In a healthy state, all functions of nervous system are carried out harmoniously. But in illness, it is upset. Our bodily organs malfunction and begin to have adverse effects on our nervous system. Major effects of illness are:

1. The threshold of visual and auditory tolerance of the nervous system often seems to be changed, e.g. when you are ill, pleasant light induces headache.
2. In illness, the reaction to stimuli may be abnormal. For examples, In amnesia, individual forgets his own kith and kin.
3. Illness affects coordination. The client often becomes irritated to do easy tasks, e.g. when client tries to walk, he/she may unable to find his balance. Concentration and thinking also affects and gives rise to complications.
4. The process of association may adversely affected. During healthy conditions, stimuli have clear and well-known meanings but is illness, they take different and strange meanings and distorted in other ways.

For example: During mania, client is confused with a well-known person.

These ideas and thoughts causes sleeplessness. This vividly affects nervous system.

In geriatric individuals, often past become real and present is disoriented in time, place and thinking.

5. Normal behavioral responses are replaced by very different responses. Some clients show the symptom of selfishness and self centered behavior.

The cause for deviated behavior may be pathological. The etiology of abnormal behavior has many complex causes and theories. The alteration in nervous system and other systems of body, psycho social causes also contributes for illness.

SENSATION AND BEHAVIOR

The information is overloaded outside of the body. That information has to reach the brain and can be used for action and responses. The information which passes into the brain through sensory organs and this process is called sensation.

Sensation is the activation of receptors in the various organs. It comprises the following.

Sensory Receptors

The sensory receptors are specialized form of neurons. These receptors are stimulated by different kinds of energy.

For example: The receptors in the eyes are triggered by light where as vibrations trigger the receptors in the ears.

Sensory Thresholds

The various sense organs like eyes, nose, ears, skin and tongue are actually quite sensitive to stimulation. According to Ernst Weber's research on determination of the smallest difference between two weights that can be detected. Its known as Weber's law of just noticeable differences (jnd or difference threshold). A jnd is the smallest difference between two stimuli that is detectable 50 percent of the time and Weber's law states that whatever the difference between stimuli might be, it is always a constant.

For example: The amount of sugar a person would need to add to a cup of tea that is already sweetened with five teaspoons is one teaspoon, then the percentage change needed to detect a just noticeable difference is 1/5 or 20 percent. If the tea has 20 teaspoons of sugar in it, the person would have to add another two teaspoons or 20 percent, to taste the difference half of the time.

Gaustar Fechner studied on absolute threshold. An absolute threshold is the smallest amount of energy needed for a person to consciously detect a stimulus 50 percent of the time it is present.
For example: sense threshold

Sight: A candle light at 30 km on a clear dark night.
Hearing: The tick of a watch 20 feet away in a quiet room.
Smell: On drop of perfume diffused throughout a three-room apartment.
Taste : One teaspoon of sugar in 9.09 liters of water.
Touch: A bee falling from 1 cm above on cheek.

Subliminal Perception

The stimuli that are below the level of conscious awareness are called subliminal stimuli. These stimuli are just strong enough to activate the sensory receptors but not strong enough for people to be consciously aware of them.

Habituation

The brain is only interested in changes in information. That's why we cannot hear the noise made in some class-rooms unless it gets very quiet. Although, they actually are hearing it, they are not paying attention to it. This is called habituation and is the way the brain deals with unchanging information.

Sensory Adaptation

The process by which constant and unchanging information from the senses of taste, touch, smell and vision is "ignored" is a different processes from habituation. The difference is that for taste, touch smell and vision, any sensory stimulus that does not change is ignored by the actual sensory receptors, not by the lower part of the brain. In sensory adaptation, the sensory receptor cells become less responsive to an unchanging stimulus.
For example: At first bite of food, mouth tastes strong at first, but as you keep eating the same thing, the taste fades out.

Physiopsychology of Sight/Seeing

Psychological properties of light

Light is a complex phenomena. Light behaves like particles as well as like waves. According to Albert Einstein, light is both, includes tiny 'packets' of waves called photons. These photons have wavelengths hence wave like properties. Light behaves in dual way. There are three psychological aspects to experience of light: brightness, color and saturation.

Brightness

It is determined by the amplitude of the wave, i.e. wave may be high or low. The higher the wave, the brighter the light will be. Low waves are dimmer. Color or hue, is determined by the length

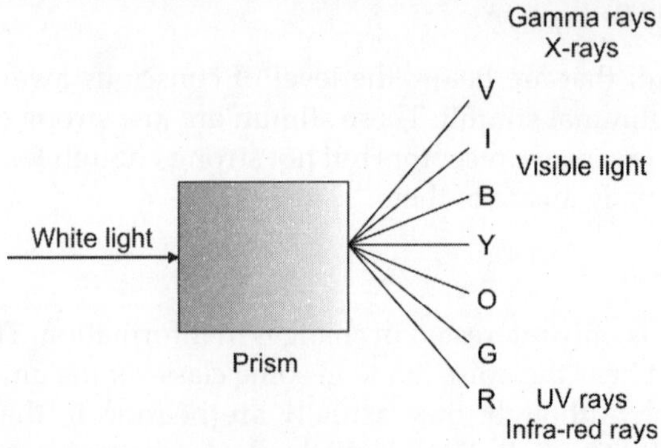

Fig. 2.4: The spectrum of light (Text book of Physiology Guyton)

of the wave. Long-wavelengths are found at the red end of the visible spectrum, whereas shorter at blue end.

Saturation: Saturation refers to the purity of the color people see. A highly saturated red, contain only red wavelengths, whereas a less saturated red might contain a mixture of wavelengths.

For example: When a child is using the red paint from a set of poster paints, the paint on the paper will look like free a pure red, but if the child mixes it in some white paint, it looks like pink. The color is still red but it will be less of a saturated red because of the presence of white wave lengths.

Structure of the Eye

The Path of Eye

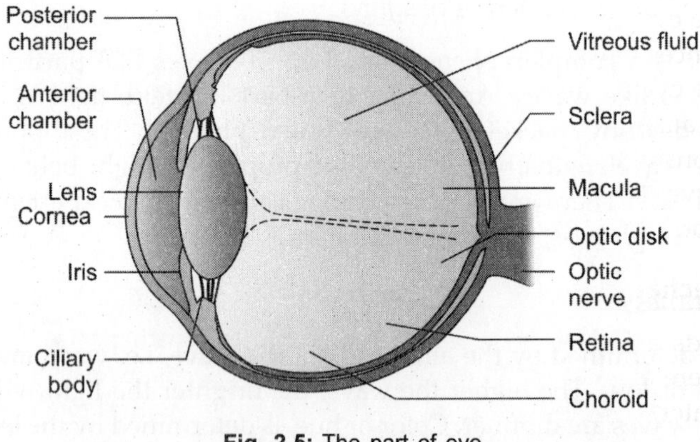

Fig. 2.5: The part of eye
(Textbook of Anatomy and Physiology Ross and Wilson)

Anatomy and Physiology of Eye

The surface of eye is covered by cornea. It protects the eye but also focuses most of the light coming into the eye. Behind it lies aqueous humor. It is a clear, watery fluid continually replenished and supplies nourishment through pupil, in a round muscle called iris. This can change the size of the pupil, letting more or less light into the eye.

Behind the iris, lies lens. It is flexible in nature and with cornea; it can change its shape from thick to thin in visual accommodation. This allows to focus on objects that are very far away or close. This property is lost in elders and lens become harder (called as presbyopia) and needs for bifocals.

Once through the lens, light passes through a large, open space filled with a clear, jelly like fluid called the vitreous humor. This also nourishes the eyes and gives it shape.

Retina, Rods and Cones

The light lastly enters the retina, a light sensitive area at the back of the eye containing three layers, ganglion cells, bipolar cells and photo receptor cells that respond to the various light waves called rods and cones. Retina contains rods and cones. It is actually receives the photons of light and turns them into neutral signals to the brain, sending them first to the bipolar cells and then to the ganglion on cells that form the optic nerve with their axons.

Blind Spot

The eyes do not adapt to constant stimuli under normal circumstances because of saccadic movements. But if people stare with one eye at one spot long-time, they may see a blank space form, because there is a "hole" in the retina—the place where all the axons of those ganglion cells leave the retina to become the optic nerve. There is no rods or cones are here, so it is referred as blind spot.

Mechanism of Eye

Rods and cones are responsible for different aspects of vision. There are about 120 million rods are found over retina except at center, where it contains cones. Rods are sensitive to changes in brightness but not to changes in wavelength, so they see only in black and white and shades of gray. They can be very sensitive because they are all lie on "party line", i.e. many rods are hooked up to only one bipolar cell, so that even only one rod is stimulated by a photon of light; the brain receives the whole area of these rods as stimulated. But because the brain does not know exactly what part of the area receiving the message, the visual acuity (sharpness) is pretty low. So, things seen in low levels of light, looks fuzzy and grayish. Because rods are located on the periphery of the retina, they are responsible for peripheral vision.

The rods function at low levels of light. Dark adaptation occurs as the eye recovers its ability to see when going from a brightly lit state to a dark state. The brighter the light was, the longer it takes the rods to adapt the new lower levels of light. This is why the bright headlights of an on coming car can leave a person less able to see for a while after the oncoming car has passed. But it is a temporary phenomenon and the rods readapt to the dark very quickly. The adaptation takes about 30 minutes and takes longer as people get older, causing night blindness in which a person strives to see well at height. Taking vitamin A supplements can relive these symptoms.

The opposite process takes into action, when going from a darkened room to one that is brightly lit. The cones have to adopt to the increased level of light, and they accomplish this light adaptation much more quickly than the rods adapt to darkness—it takes a few seconds at most. There are about 6 million cones on each eye, of these 50,000 have a private line to the optic nerve, i.e. cones found in the very center of the retina in an area called the fovea, are the receptors for visual acuity. It also means that the cones need a lot more light to function than the rods do, so cones works in bright light. Cones are also sensitive to different wave lengths of tight, so they are responsible for color vision.

Color Blindness

It is caused by defective cones in the retina of the eye. It is one set of cones is inherited in a pattern known as sex-linked inheritance, much more inherited in men than women. Men can inherit it from their mother's X-chromosome only, whereas women must inherit two defective genes to be color blind.

The Hearing Sense

Physiopsychology of Hearing

The properties of sound are similar to light but differs in physical properties. Sound waves are the vibrations of the molecules of air that surround us. Sound waves have wavelengths, amplitude and purity. The wavelengths are interpreted by the brain as the frequency or pitch. Pitch may be high, low or medium. Amplitude is interpreted as volume how soft or loud a sound is. The saturation of sound is called timbre, richness in the tones of the sound. Many pure tones cannot be heard in day to day because of noise.

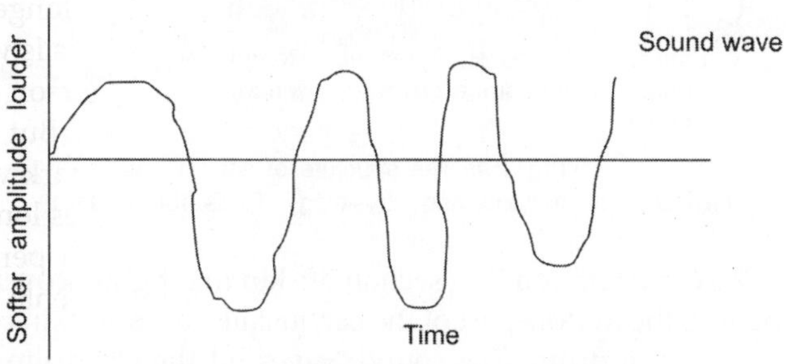

Fig. 2.6: The structure of sound wavelengths (Textbook of Anatomy and Physiology Guyton)

As the person's vision is limited to spectrum of light, he is also limited to sound frequencies of sound. Frequency of sound is measured in hertz (Hz). Human ear can hear between 20 and 20,000 Hz, most accurate hearing occurs at 1,000 Hz.

Anatomy and Physiology of Ear

The ear is a series of structures, each of which plays a part in hearing. The 8th cranial nerve or vestibulo cochlear nerve supplies the ear. The ear is divided into 3 parts. 1. External/ outer ear, 2. The middle ear or tympanic cavity, 3. Inner/Internal ear.

External Ear/Outer Ear

The pinna is the visible, external part of the ear that functions as a concentrator, funneling the sound waves from outside into the structure of ear. It is an entrance to the auditory canal (ear canal), the short tunnel that runs down to the tympanic membrane or ear

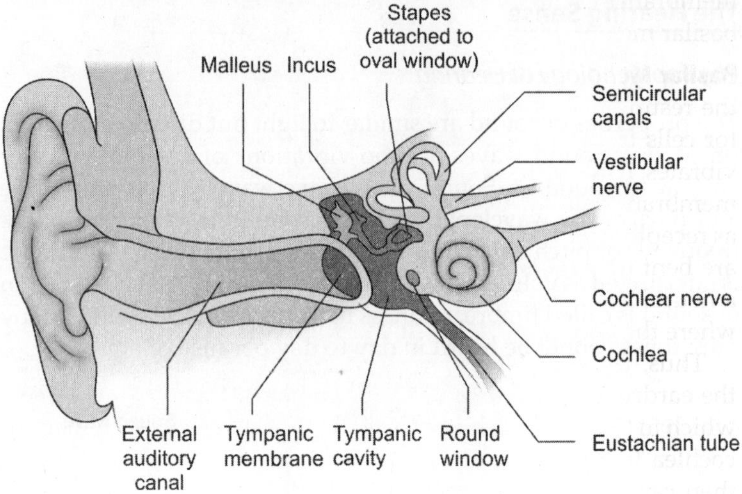

Fig. 2.7: The structure of ear
(Textbook of Anatomy and Physiology Ross and Wilson)

drum. The ear drum is a thin section of skin that tightly covers the opening into the middle part of the ear, just like a drum skin covers the opening in a drum. The sound waves hit the ear drum, as it vibrates and causes three tiny bones in the middle ear to vibrate.

Middle Ear

The three small bones are known as auditory ossicles and individually as the hammer, anvil and stirrup. When the ear drum vibrates, the hammer resting against the eardrum also vibrates causing a chain reaction in the anvil and the stirrup. As the vibrations travel down the bones, they are amplified to certain extent. The stirrup, the last bone in the chain, rests against another membrane of tissue called the oval window, which in turn covers the entrance to the inner ear.

Inner Ear

The oval window vibrates when the stirrup vibrates, setting up a chain reaction in the inner ear.

Cochlea: The inner ear is a snail- shaped structure called the cochlea, which is filled with fluid. When the oval window vibrates, it causes the fluid in the cochlea to vibrate. This fluid surrounds a membrane running thorough the middle of the cochlea called the basilar membrane.

Basilar Membrane and Organ of Corti: The basilar membrane is the resting place of the organ of corti, which contains the receptor cells from the sense of hearing. When the basilar membrane vibrates, it vibrates the organ of corti, causing it to brush against a membrane above it. On the organ of corti, lies hair cells which acts as receptors for sound. When these auditory receptors or hair cells are bent up against the other membrane, it causes them to send a neural message through the auditory nerve and into the brain, where the auditory cortex will interpret the sounds.

Thus, the sound waves go in through the pinna and vibrate the eardrum, which then vibrates the hammer, anvil and stirrup, which in turn vibrate the oval window. This causes the fluid in the cochlea to vibrate, which vibrates the basilar membrane, which then causes the organ corti to move up and bend its hair cells, which send signals about hearing to the brain. Of course, the louder the sound in the outside world, the stronger the vibrations that stimulate more of these hair cells, which the brain interprets as loudness.

Types of Hearing Impairments

Hearing impairment is the term used to refer to difficulties in hearing. A person can be partially or totally hearing impaired and the management of treatment varies according to the reason for the impairment. There are 2 types of hearing impairment.

Conduction Hearing Impairment: It can result from either a damaged eardrum or damage to the bones of the middle ear. In the latter case, sounds cannot be conducted from the eardrum to the cochlea. Middle ear damage is often from ear infections that are not treated quickly enough or from chronic ear infections. In this case, use of hearing aids helps to restore the hearing.

Nerve Hearing Impairment: In this impairment, the problem lies either in the inner ear or in the auditory pathways and cortical areas of the brain. By adulthood, half of hair cells are lost. Exposure to loud noises, cause hair cells to break and speed up this loss, resulting in earlier hearing problems.

Nerve hearing impairment cannot be helped by ordinary hearing aids because of nerve involvement. These are basically sound amplifiers. Cochlear implantation helps to restore the hearing loss in these clients. Cochlear implant bypasses the outer and middle ears by sending signals from a microphone worn behind ear to a sound processor worn on the belt or in a pocket, which then translates those signals into electrical stimuli that are sent to a series of electrodes implanted directly into the brain. The brain then processes the electrode information as sound. With an implant, people can hear some speech and their own speech to a degree that allows more communication with others. In this aspect, client should be counseled about the therapeutic use of implants.

SENSE OF TASTE

The sense of taste includes a combination of taste and smell.

GUSTATION (Sensation of Taste)

Taste Buds

The receptors for the sensation of taste are called taste buds. These are found in the papillae of the tongue and are widely distributed in the epithelium of the tongue, soft palate, pharynx and epiglottis.

The tongue of an adult nearly contains 10,000 taste buds. Each bud is a oval structure which consists of three kinds of epithelial cells. They are the gustatory receptor cells, supporting cells and the basal cells. Each taste bud contains about forty taste receptor cells, that extend into a tiny opening in the epithelium of the taste bud, called a taste pore. Taste buds are found in elevation, of the tongue called papillae. They are circum vallate papillae, fungifrom and filiform papillae.

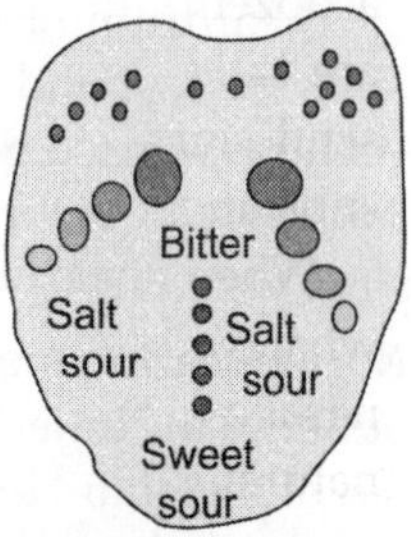

Fig. 2.8: Various sensations in tongue (Textbook of Anatomy and Physiology Ross and Wilson)

Each taste bud has about 20 receptors and acts like a neuron at synapse site. They receive molecules of various substances that fit into the receptor sites like key into a lock.

Taste is usually called as chemical reactions with the molecules of food is first dissolved in saliva. Then it mixes with taste hairs that extend into the taste pores and initiate action potentials. These action potentials are propagated as taste impulse which passes through the facial, glossophyrageal and vagus nerves. The nerve impulses are transmitted to the thalamus, then to the primary taste area in the parietal lobe of the cerebral cortex, one in each hemisphere, where the taste is received. We have four types of sensation of taste. They are sweet, sour, bitter and salt. If any injury occurs to buds, they are replaced and carry works out mechanism.

We feel less tasty of food when we have cold. It is because, we can taste only sweet, salty, bitter sour and umami and nose is packed with cold, so, we do not get enhanced variations of those tastes that come from the sense of smell.

In 1996, Lindemann postulated that there is fifth kind of taste receptor that detects a pleasant "brothy" taste associated with foods like cheese, soyabean, chicken soup. He called this as "Umami" which translates the Japanese word to describe the taste. These five taste sensations work together, along with the sense of smell and the texture, temperature and 'heat" of foods, to produce many more of taste sensations.

OLFACTION (The sense of smell)

The ability to smell odors is called olfaction or olfactory sense. Actually, people do not smell from nose. The outer part of nose is just a transmitter. It receives the odors and translates into neural signals. These are situated at the top of nasal passages. This area of olfactory receptor cells is only about an inch square in each cavity probably contains 10 million olfactory receptors.

The olfactory receptor cells each have about a half dozen to a dozen little 'hairs', that project into the cavity. These "hairs" are called 'cilia'. There are receptor sites as these hair cells that send signals to the brain when stimulated by the molecules of substances that are in the air moving past them.

When a person is sniffing, it serves to move molecules of whatever the person is trying to smell into the nose and into the nasal cavities. Olfactory receptors also have to be replaced as they naturally die off, about every 5 to 8 weeks. There are more than five types of olfactory receptors. In fact, there are at least 1000 of them. In brain, the olfactory center which modulates the olfactory bulbs.

The olfactory bulbs are located right on top of the sinus cavity on each side of the brain directly beneath the frontal lobes. (Fig. 2.9). The olfactory receptors send their neural signals

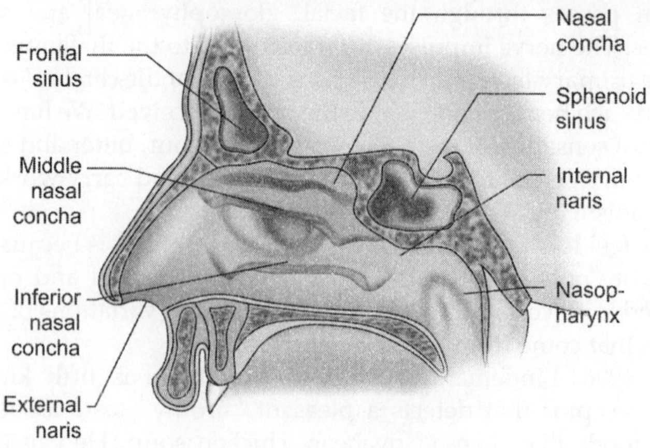

Fig. 2.9: The sense of smell
(Textbook of Anatomy and Physiology Ross and Wilson)

directly up to these bulbs, bypassing the entire lower brain and its selective attention filter, the reticular formation. People can ignore a smell that is constant and unchanging, but it does not involve the reticular formation.

Sense of Touch (Somesthetic Senses)

The sense of touch includes many sensations, originating in different places in and on the body. These senses can be called as somesthetic senses. The word 'soma' refers to 'the body' and 'esthetic' means feeling. There are three somesthetic sense systems, the skin senses, the kinesthetic sense and vestibular senses. The skin senses do with touch, pressure, temperature and pain. The kinesthetic sense do with the location of body parts in relation to ground and to each other, whereas, the vestibular senses functions in relation to movement and body position.

Feeling of Touch, Pressure and Temperature

The skin is an organ. The site of skin approximately is about 20 square feet. It functions to bodily fluids in and germs out, receives and transmits information from the outside world to the central nervous nervous system (somato sensory cortex). The information

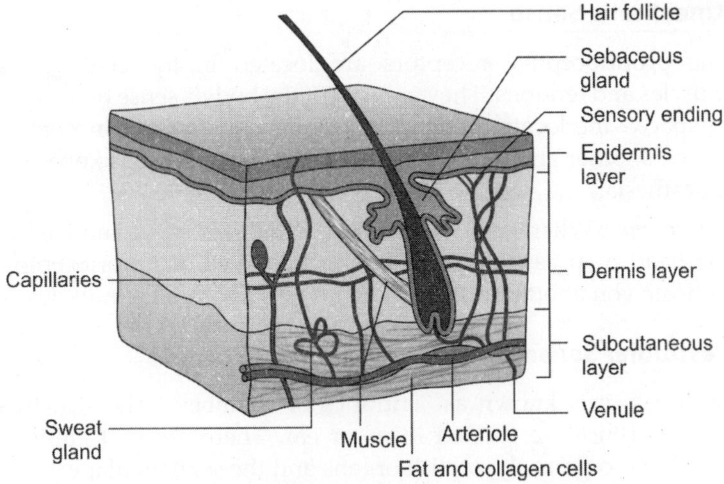

Fig. 2.10: Cross-section of skin and receptors (Textbook of Anatomy and Physiology Ross and Wilson)

about light touch, deeper pressure, hot, cold, and pain is colleated by special receptors in the skin layers.

Sensory Receptors

There are about a half dozen different receptors in the layers of the skin (Fig. 2.10).

Some of them will respond to only one kind of sensation, e.g. the Pacinian corpuscles are just beneath the skin and respond to pressure only. To this, nerve endings are wrapped around the ends of the hair follicles. These are sensitive to both pain and touch. There are free nerve endings just beneath the uppermost layer of the skin that respond to changes in temperature and to pressure and to pain.

There are pain fibers in the internal organs as well as receptors for pressure, e.g. hitting from a hammer on thumb. Primly, feelings of sharp bright and fast and later the bruised issue simply aches. Feeling pain in stomach. Actually, there are different types of pain. There are proprioceptive receptors that detect pain and pressure in the organs, e.g. visceral pain but pain sensations in the skin, muscles, tendons and joints are carried on large nerve fibers are called somatic pain. This somatic pain acts as a kind of reminder system, keeping people from further injury by reminding them that the body has already been damaged.

Kinesthetic Sense

The proprioceptive receptors are located in the skin, joints, muscles and tendons. They are part of the body's sense of position in space—the location of the arms, legs and so forth in relation to one another and to the ground. This type of sense is known as kinesthesia.

For example: When you close your eyes and raise your hand above the head, you can locate your hand because of proprioceptors indicate you about the changes in pressure within the muscles.

Vestibular Sense

In Greek, it is known as "entrance or chamber". The structure for this sense are located in inner ear. There are two kinds of vestibular organs, the otolith organs and the semicircular canals.

The otolith organs are tiny sacs found just above the cochlea. These sacs contain a gelation like fluid within which tiny crystals are suspended. The head moves and the crystals also moves or vibrates, setting off some tiny hair like receptors on the inner surface of the sac, telling the person that the he or she is moving forward, back, round, sideways or up and down.

The semicircular canals are three in number tubes that are also filled with fluid and will stimulate hair like receptors when rotated. There are three tubes so that there is one each of the three planes of motion. Within these three planes, the body rotates, it sets off the receptors in these canals. Imbalance in these proportions leads to dizziness and vomiting.

For example: Motion sickness.

The Glands and Psychology

Glands are the organs in the body that secrete chemicals. Some glands namely salivary glands secrete their chemicals directly onto the body's tissues through ducts. The ductless glands or endocrine glands secrete the hormones. They pass directly to the blood stream. A hormone is a chemical messenger secreted by an endocrine gland and carried through the blood to act on target organ or tissue. The internal functions of the body is controlled and regulated partly by hormones and partly by autonomic nervous system. The hormones affect behavior and emotions by controlling muscles and organs. Emotional state that the surge in certain hormones actually triggers the emotional reaction. The endocrine glands are:

a. Pituitary gland – 1
b. Thyroid gland – 1
c. Parathyroid gland – 4
d. Adrenal (Supra renal) glands and - 2 islets of langerhan's of pancreases.
e. Pineal gland or body – 1
f. Ovaries in the female – 2
g. Testes in the male – 2.

Pituitary/Master Gland

It is located in hypothalamus of the brain. This hypothalamus controls the glandular system by influencing the pituitary. So it is called master gland, the one that controls or influences all of the other endocrine glands.

Thyroid Gland

The thyroid gland is located inside the neck and secretes a hormone called thyroxin (T3 and T4) that regulates the metabolism of the body.

Pineal Gland

It is located in the brain, nearer to the back. It secretes a hormone called melatonin, which regulate the sleep wake cycle.

Pancreas

Pancreas secrete the hormone insulin and glucagon which regulates the blood sugar in the body. The deficient secretion leads diabetes, where as excessive secretion results in hypoglycemia or low blood sugar, which causes the individual to feel always hungry and thirsty and often become overweight as a result.

Gonads

These are situated one on top of each kidney. It is divided into adrenal medulla and the adrenal cortex. Adrenal medulla secretes epinephrine and norepinepherine when individual are under stress and anxiety and that aids in sympathetic arousal.

The adrenal cortex produces over 30 different hormones called corticoids or steroids that regulates salt intake and stress reaction. It also provides a source of sex hormones to those provided by the gonads. The hormone cortisol is released when individual faces stress. Cortisol is important in the release of glucose into the blood stream during stress, providing energy for the brain itself and the release of fatty acids from the fat cells that provide the muscles with energy.

Apart from these hormones are recently several hormones discovered. These are called growth factors. They act locally as autocrines or paracrines. Overall, for normal behavior all the endocrine as well as exocrine glands has to perform harmoniously. Any deviation in production and action can results in abnormality of behavior.

GLANDS AND NURSING PERCEPTIVE

The knowledge of sense organs and glands helps to know the client in a comprehensive way. The nurse has to know the following:

1. There is a relationship between the functioning of sense organs, glands and muscular system with emotional states. Positive emotions encourage normal flow of fluids whereas negative emotions and stress causes altered (hyper or hypo) secretion of fluids. So, nurse has to comprehend the relation between these systems.
2. As far as possible, nurse has to avoid in the sick room the negative emotions which cause stress and strain to clients

which it itself alters the body mechanism. Nurses etiquettes, good nature, sympathy, cheerfulness brings a healthy emotional tone to the atmosphere in the patient's wards.

3. Nurses in the wards suffers from burnout and desk rage symptoms. Always, she comes in contact with suffering, negative emotional state, depression and death. Patient's nature will be varied. So, nurses have to seek an outlet for her anxiety. Involvement in recreation, hobbies, friendships, humor clubs, yoga, which is a medium for self expression and helps to maintain the balance between mind and body.

Nature of Behavior

Behavior is an integrated complex process. But, the question arises that whether behavior is nature made or environment (nurture). In 17th century, British philosopher John Locke believed that the mind of a newborn infant is a "blank slate" (tabularasa). What gets written on this slate is what the baby experiences—what he or she sees, hears, tastes, smells and feels. According to Locke, all knowledge comes us through our senses. It is provided by experience no knowledge or ideas are built in.

In the 19th century Darwin, theory and behaviorists such as John B Watson and BF Skinner postulated that human nature is completely malleable. Early training can turn a child into any kind of adult, regardless of his or her heredity.

Today's newer psychologists agree not only both nature and nurture play important roles but they interact continuously to guide the development of behavior.

Summary Points

- Mind is a complex phenomena which includes conscious subconscious and unconscious.
- Mind and body are always interacted. They are the same faces of a coin.
- The nervous system is a complex network of cells that carries information to and from all parts of the body.
- The central nervous system consists of brain and spinal cord.
- The peripheral nervous system contains somatic nervous system and the autonomic nervous system.
- Brain contains medulla, pons, cerebrum and cerebellum.

- The thalamus is the switching station that sends sensory information to the cortex.
- The hypothalamus controls hunger, thirst, sleep, sexual behavior and waking emotions. It also controls pituitary gland.
- The limbic system consists of the thalamus, hypothalamus, hippocampus, amygdala and fornix.
- The hippocampus is responsible for storing memories and remembering location of objects.
- The amygdala controls fear responses and memory of fearful stimuli.
- Endocrine glands secrete hormones directly into the blood stream, influencing the activity of the muscles and organs.

Test Yourself

1. Discuss mind-body interaction.
2. Define neuron, Explain the structure and functions of neuron.
3. Explain the roles of inheritance in psychological development.
4. What are the sense organs? Explain the functions of the sense organs.
5. List out the different endocrine glands.
6. Elaborate the importance of muscles in nursing.
7. Discuss nature versus nurture in psychological development.

Chapter 3

Cognition, Attention, Perception, Learning, Memory, Thinking, Intelligence

ATTENTION

Always our sense organs bombarded with external stimuli. But we perceive very few to our knowledge. Perceiving and attending to certain selective stimuli is known as attention. Attention is the perceptual processes that select certain inputs for inclusion in our conscious experience or awareness at any given moment.

Attention is not a fixed state of mind. It is an activity which grows and changes. It is constantly shifting from one object to another or from one aspect of another situation.

Attention involves motor adjustments, which the individual has to make in the process of attention. It is a sort of psychomotor activity which we have so adjust muscles and senses so that they are concentrated on a limited portion of object or environment.

DETERMINANTS OF ATTENTION

The following factors contribute for attention:

a. *Intensity of stimuli:* Overall, the strong stimulus will attract more quickly than a weak, shabby one-large size, loud sounds, bright colors and light attracts our attention.
b. *Quantity of stimuli:* If the stimuli remain constant over a long period, it attracts than moving temporary stimuli, e.g. working clock may not attract our attention but if it stops, it attracts our attention.
c. *Movement:* On the whole, moving things attracts heavily than stationary objects.

For example: fast moving motor cycle with loud noise attracts our attention than normal speed vehicles.

d. *Size:* Large scale attracts more than tiny ones. But, if there is a very small object against a large or huge background, it will attract our attention. We usually view the tall or very small persons.
e. *Contrast:* Any object that is strikingly different from its surroundings will tend to stand out and attract attention, e.g. a black spot on a white shirt.
f. *Repetition*: A moving, repeated objects attracts our attention, e.g. a repeated cry or sign.

Types of Attention

Attention varies according to situations and mental make up. It can be involuntary, voluntary or habitual. At times, may be partially involuntary and partially voluntary or habitual.

In involuntary attention, persons attend to an object or a stimulus against our 'will' because of its unique striking qualities. *For example*: When we hear an abnormally, loud sound, we jump out to see while writing also. Because the loud sound captures our attention. We attend to those stimuli naturally easily or spontaneously without any effort of will. We yield to the stimulus.

Sometimes, we have to deliberately direct our attention to a stimulus or situation. We have to make a conscious effort to do so. This is known as voluntary attention. It is not spontaneous in nature. It needs more efforts and time.

For example: Learning difficult lessons. Voluntary attention becomes easy if some interest is created during the process of attending to an uninteresting task. If we give more voluntary attention to a subject for long-time, it results in boring and irritation.

In habitual attention, there is no conscious effort or sensation to attract our involuntary any attention. We perceive them because of our attitudes, habits or interests, e.g. attention given to nursing procedure.

The span of attention: The maximum amount of material that can be attended to in one period of attention is called, 'span of attention'.

For example: If you notice six digits or letters in a single act of attention, your span of attention six.

Distraction of attention refers to shifting of attention from one stimulus to another frequently.

Division of attention: It refers to the process of dividing or attention equally and simultaneously between two or more objects. *For example*: Listening to movie songs and writing assignment. The division of attention leads to the deterioration of quality and quantity of all the tasks attended simultaneously.

For example: Internal distraction: Thoughts, pain, headache.

External distraction: Noise, bright light.

Alteration in Attention

The deviation in the process of attention is known as distraction. It may be continuous or discontinuous.

Continuous Distraction

A stimulus interfering in attention for a long periods is called continuous distraction, e.g. noise of a train.

Discontinuous Distraction

When a stimuli distracts the person's attention with certain time is called discontinuous distraction, e.g. lights off.

Distraction affects the quantity and quality of performance. In much noise, students cannot memorize the material. However, the research found that discontinuous distracter create more affect on performance than continuous distracter. The research show that during the process of distraction , muscular activity of person increases and the person do the task with more speed but makes more mistakes and errors. Age, health conditions, nature of task also alters the attention span. In children, if attention span lacks in quantity and quality for a certain period, it leads to attention deficit disorders.

PERCEPTION

Information enters into the body through senses by bits and pieces but it is not actual what we perceive. The people perceive the world of objects and people, a world that bombards us with integrated wholes, not piecemeal sensations.

Perception is the study of how we integrate sensory information into percepts of objects and how we then use these percepts to get around in the world.

According to Meyer E. Glenn-Perception is the method by which people take all the sensations they experience at any given moment and interpret them in some meaningful fashion.

Constancies: Size, Shape and Brightness

Size Constancy: It is the tendency to interpret an object as always being the same size, regardless of its distance from the viewer, if an object that is normally perceived to be about six feet tall appears very small on the retina it will be interpreted as being very for away, e.g. six month old infants.

Size constancy cannot be fully present at birth or it must require some stimulation from outer environment.

Shape Constancy

It is the shape of the object as constant, even when it changes on the retina. This is called shape constancy and is why a person still perceives a coin as a circle even if it is held at an angle that makes it appear to be an oval on the retina. Another example that dinner plates on a table are also seen as round, even though from the angle of viewing they are oval.

Brightness Constancy

This is the tendency to perceive the apparent brightness of an object as the same even when the light conditions change.

For example: If a person is wearing black pants and a white shirt, in a day the shirt will appear to be much brighter than the pants. But if the sun is covered by thick clouds, even though the pants and shirt have less light to reflect than previously, the shirt will still appear brighter than the pants as before, because of the different amount of light reflected from each piece of clothing is still the same difference as before.

PRINCIPLES OF PERCEPTION

Perception is affected by different factors. These are classified broadly as:

1. Gestalt law of organization
2. Subjective factors
3. Objective factors.

Gestalt law of organization

The image projected on our retina is a mosaic of varying brightness and colors. Somehow our perceptual system organizes the mosaic into a set of discrete objects projected against a background. This was the idea of Gestalt psychology. Gestalt psychology theorists emphasized the importance of perceiving whole objects or forms, and proposed a number of principles of how we organize objects.

Figure Ground Relationships

In a stimulus that contains two or more distinct regions, we usually see a part of it as a figure and the rest as ground. The regions seen as a figure contain the objects of interest they appear more solid than the ground and appear in front of the ground. This is the most elementary form of perceptual organization.

Necker Cube: It is a reversible and ambiguous figure. Since it is not clear which pattern should predominate.

Figure Ground: What it depicts? Is it a wine glass? Or two faces looking each other. This is an example in which the figure and the ground seem to "Switch" each time you look at the picture.

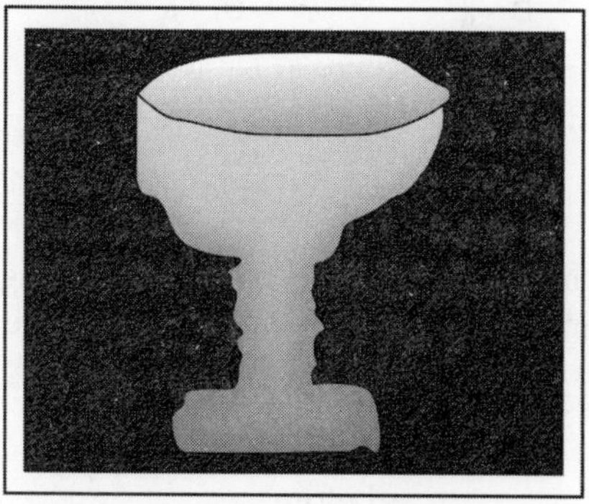

Fig. 3.1: Ground relationships (Reference: Psychology - MUNN and Munn)

Proximity or Nearness

It is the tendency to perceive objects that are close to one another as part of the same grouping.

For example: The below circles will be perceived as two lines of circles.

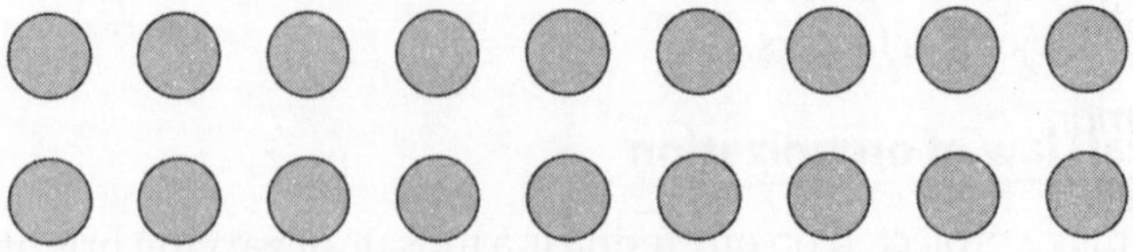

Similarity (Reference : Psychology - MUNN and Munn)

It refers to the tendency to perceive things that look similar as being part of the same group.

For example: Wearing same uniform in sports to highlight the group.

Closure

It is the tendency to complete figures that are incomplete.

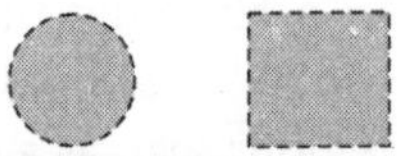

For example: Drawing curved lines spaced in apart in a circular pattern on board. They look like a circle but really its not. They are just curved lines laid out in a circular fashion. The brain fills the gaps between the arcs to perceive a circle.

Continuity

It refers to the tendency to perceive things as possible with a continuous pattern rather than with a complex, broken up pattern.

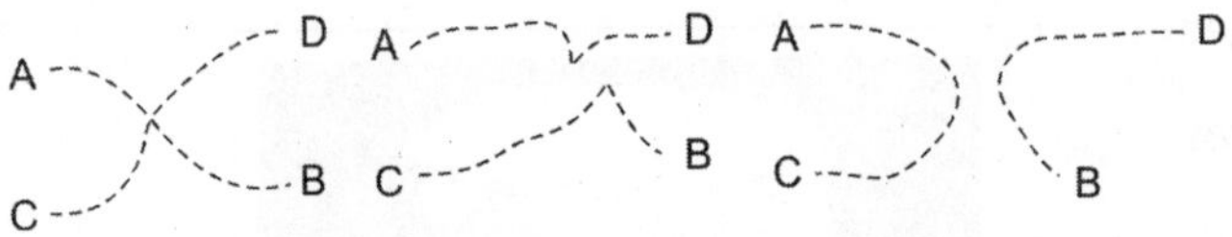

Contiguity

Contiguity is the tendency to perceive two things that happen close together in time as being related. Usually the first occurring event is seen as causing the second event.

Inclusion

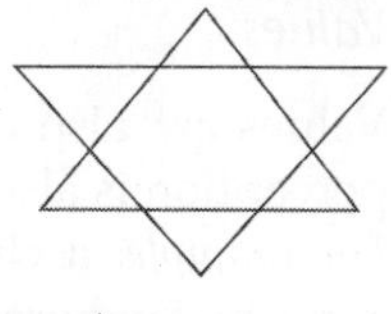

In this perception, any figure or form is not perceived in parts but the parts are organized in perception best possible whole form.

In this figure, two inverted triangles looks like a star.

Common Fate

It is related to movement. If some stimuli are moving in one direction are perceived as a unit perception, e.g. trees titled in one direction because of speed of wind are perceived as one in perception.

Subjective Factors

Perception is also depends upon certain organismic factors of the internal characteristics of a person. Because of subjectivity in perceiving, individuals differ in determining the affect.

Mental set

It means psychological preparedness can also affect the perception. *For example:* Memorizing certain questions and answers during examinations gets very fast.

Motives and Needs

- Motives of an individual do affect the perception.

For example: An interested person in certain learning subjects learns faster than others.

- Needs also determine the perception.
  For example: a man in need for money listens and searches for getting it as early as possible.

Interest

Interest in particular subject also contributes for perception.

For example: A cricket crazy person listens the latest score with attentively.

Emotions

Emotional state often contributes for perception.
For example: at night, fine sounds are also heard very easily.

Values

Values are also contributes for many happenings around us. So perception is also greatly affected by it.
For example: a child of alcoholic father will perceive alcohol as a normal where as child belonging to orthodoxy family may perceive it as abnormal and harmful.

Habits

Habits can also affect the perception. Habits direct perception in a particular way. A person with white apron usually we perceive him as a doctor/nurse/health personnel, because it is our habit to view them in white dresses.

Familiarity

Those stimuli with which there is good familiarity can be recognized from far away distances. We can recognize our parents and kith and kins from far distances and even in dim light situations.

Attitude

Attitudes toward others can also influences perception about them. If a person has favorable attitude toward drinking, he will ignore any information points towards its harmfulness.

Past Experiences

Good or bitter experiences of past influence perception. A child bitten by a dog in childhood will perceive all dogs as dangerous. However, good/ sweet experiences also favors perception in a positive way. A child experienced a very kind stranger will perceive strangers as nice and good people.

Objective Factors

Objective external characteristics of stimulus shows affect on perception. The size, intensity, color, contrast, rareness, novelty, suddenness, movement, etc. also affect our perception.

PERCEPTUAL ERRORS

Abnormalities in perception may be temporary or permanent because of defect in sense organs. Sensation is the vehicle through which perception is perceived. Any defect in sense organs like cataract, people experience difficulty in identifying objects.

Sensory deprivation also contributes for error in perception. Long-term sensory deprivation leads to abnormal perception. Early experience after birth have long lasting effect on perception.

Environmental factors also contribute for error in perception. This is known as illusion. Illusion is a perception that does not correspond to reality. In darkness, we perceive a rope as a snake. Fatigue and sickness can also cause error in perception.

In Müller-Lyer illusion, the distortion happens when the viewer tries to determine if the two lines are exactly the same length. They are identical, but one line looks longer the other. The reason is that most people live in a world with many of buildings. Buildings have corners. When a person is outside a building, the corner of the building is close to that person, while the walls seem to be moving away. When the person is inside a building, the corner of the room seems to move away from the viewer while the walls are coming closer. In the illusion, the line with the angles facing inward is like the outside of the building, and the one with the angles facing outward is like the inside of the room. In their minds, people "pull" the inward-facing angles toward them like the outside corners of a building and they make the outward facing angles 'stretch' away from them like the outside corners of the room.

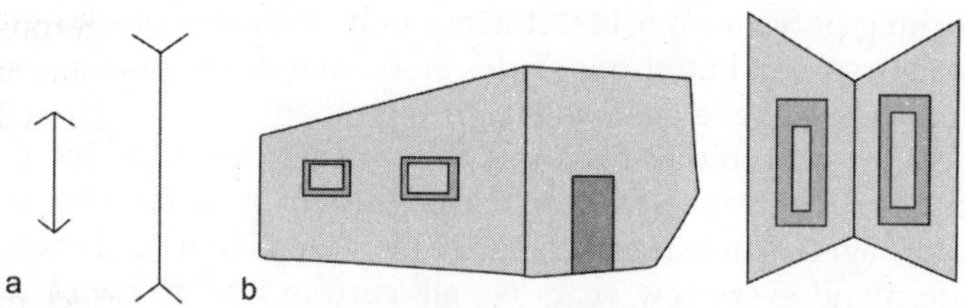

Fig. 3.2: Müller-Lyer illusion (Reference: Psychology; Munn and Munn)

One more common illusion is moon illusion. In this, the moon on the horizon appears to be much larger than the moon in the sky.

The other altered perception is of motion. Sometimes people perceive an object as moving when it is really still. Another illusion related to motion is stroboscopic motion is closed phi phenomenon. In this, lights turned on in sequence appear to move.

For example: If a light is turned on in a darkened room and then turned off and then another light a short-distance away is flashed on and off, it will appear to be one light moving across that distance.

The other main error in perception is delusion. It is a false belief that cannot be modified by reasoning or by demonstration of facts. These are seen in psychoses. These delusions chronically affect the perception of person. *For example:* If client is suffering from delusion of persecution, will perceive that people are harming him and spying about him. Because of this false belief, he may attack on others.

Another abnormality in perception is hallucination. It is a total false perception. In this, client accepts the imaginary things as real, but in reality they do not exist. *For example:* Client may hear sounds but in reality, it may not exist. The cause may be physio-psychological, such as chronic drinking, drug abuse, etc. These symptoms are seen in chronic cases of mentally ill such as schizophrenia, Manic depressive psychoses and alcoholism. The knowledge of nurse on physio-psychological process of perception helps for understanding the mentally ill and can deliver an evidence based care.

LEARNING

Learning pervades our life. It is not only acquiring or mastering the new subject but also includes emotional development, social interaction and even personality development.

We learn everyday from our lives. Babies learn to kick their legs to move, teenagers learn the rhymes of their favorite ones, middle aged people learn to change their food habits and exercise pattern and every few years we all learn to find a new style of cosmetics go out of fashion. This shows that learning is not always intentional.

Learning: Definition

In a broad way, learning occurs when experience causes a relatively permanent change in an individual's behavior or knowledge. The change may be deliberate or unintentional, for better or worse, correct or incorrect, and conscious or unconscious (Hill, 2002). To qualify on learning, this change must be brought about by experience by the interaction of a person with his or her environment. Changes simply caused by maturation such as growing taller or becoming white hair, do not qualify the act of learning.

According to Skinner, "Learning is not acquiring knowledge or skill by mere mechanical repetitions. It is a process in which the learner organizes different elements and experiences to reach a particular goal."

In the view of Hilgard, learning refers to the change in a subject's behavior to a given situation brought about by his repeated experiences in that situation, provided that the behavior change cannot be explained on the basis of native response tendencies, maturation or temporary states of the subject.

In the opinion of kingley and Gray "Learning is the process by which an organism is satisfying its motivation adopts and adjusts its behavior in order to overcome obstacles or barriers."

Blair Jones and Simpson are of the view that "any change of behavior which is a result of experience and which causes people to face later situations differently may be called learning.

Gutherie in "psychology of learning" "says" "the ability to learn, that is, to respond differently to a situation because of past response to the situation".

According to EC Tolman, "Learning is the name given to a small number of demonstrable relationships between environmental factors (stimuli) and behavioral changes (responses).

Learning may be considered finally as the process of constant change or modifications of behavior through continual interaction with the environment by the individuals. It is an integral or overall aspect of the individuals development in its widest sense.

Nature of Learning

Man learns and also trains others. *For example:* In circus, elephant does many tricks. The animals can do some aspects of what man do but not in language skills. It is because, the vocal center of animals lacks what human being possess. Human beings can read, write, play, make TV, computer, bomb, etc. and can gather information about it but not animals. This complex knowledge, the animals cannot acquire. Mind of human beings is a developed one and that is why are able to master the knowledge of higher level. What learning does for a human and how it affects can be viewed as follows:

1. Learning is modification of behavior: Learning produces change in behavior. Learning is often defined as the modification of behavior. The child learns ideas, rules and regulations, customs, values, traditions, etc. from his surrounding environment and for different complex situations in life. So, the individual displays the required behavior and predicted activities, though no one teaches him to do so. Gradually this modification of behavior becomes permanent and goes on developing and changing day by day.

2. Learning helps to reach the motto: Learning not only brings change in behavior but also helps one in meeting his desires. Goals and ambition can be achieved only by appropriate learning in a particular defined direction. It directly or indirectly helps the individual to reach his goal. Learning of speech, laugh, cry, in child is organized deliberately. They are not accidental. Hence, learning is accepted by all as an intentional process.

3. Learning creates interest to know new things: A deep interest for knowledge helps to find out new facts and engage himself in research. This helps to learn more and more. Learning leads to happiness and in turn it activates for new learning.

4. Environmental influence brings difference in learning: All children grow in different environments. Learning process and its effect on one child is different from that of another on the basis of their difference in environment in which their learning experience takes places. Children from adverse conditions, such as poverty, sometimes show a glorious result in learning. So also those coming from a proper environment sometimes show the same originality in learning. Children from unfavorable conditions fail to become successful in learning due to their poor back up. On the other side, children in bigger cities, inspite of their low intelligence, prove successful in showing better in learning. This is because of their environment helps to mould them to learn better. Hence, we can conclude that a proper and adequate environment is very much necessary for a fruitful learning of the child. Primly the home and school should provide adequate stimulus to experience the learning.

5. Learning is a problem solving activity: The society is complex and dynamic. Individual has to adjust to changing faces of society. He has to face many novel and unwarned situations.

There are some problems that cannot be solved by means of age old customary methods. The novel situations should be met with new ideas and at this point learning help him. New learning helps to solve the complex problems.

6. Learning is a master of habit: Habits are formed by repetition of work. Learning is the display of mastered personal reaction to a given situation. Man has to react in the right way to his stimulus. By habit formation, he can do with incorrect ways of reaction formation. Secondly learning makes habit not only be formed in the correct way but also organized.

7. Learning is automatic process: Learning takes place when the child becomes active. He has to indulge himself in the process of learning. In course of performing daily activities he automatically gathers experiences. Experience makes him to learn and to know the future requirements psychological, social, emotional and cultural, etc. he becomes active to capture it. His requirements, stimulate his will and produces response. If he is easily motivated by some other factors, then learning can also take place even without a tutor. The child learns when he feels the requirements for it. So this process is always directed to a particular goal.

8. Learning is not knowledge about subjects: Only reading or studying in schools or colleges is not learning. All round development of child is learning and by only one's personality matures. Apart from study subjects, knowledge about art, literature, philosophy, God, reality, social values, personal traits also learned by people. So, it should not be mean that learning implies only reading text books.

9. Learning may be correct or incorrect: Learning should be socially acceptable or unacceptable. Real learning warns us against bad behaviors.

10. Learning may be formal and informal: Learning is from womb to tomb. Child learns many things from social interaction with others in his environment. New habits are formed and skills mastered. Many novel ideas also occur to his own mind. New choices, new beliefs and interests are aroused in him. Then he enters the school and learns what teachers has taught. He knows what he is learning. These all are termed as formal learning. Apart from these, he also learns informally by agencies such as home, social club, gatherings, religious places, play ground, exercusion and on field, etc. render informal learning to him.

11. Higher learning depends upon capacity of individual and complexity of learning material: Many factors contribute for successful learning, they are at individual levels such as memory thinking, motivation, understanding, emotion controlling capacity and many more. To make learning effective, the child takes help of two processes. One is that he tries to solve some of his problems with already acquired knowledge and skill and the second is that he discovers new methods and skills to face some personal problems. In order to solve complex problems he needs higher learning.

12. Learning is function of maturation: Learning to an extent is also a function of maturation, one cannot teach a neonate to walk, his sensory motor and also nervous system including brain must reach a certain level of maturity. The predetermined sequential stage of maturity of the sensory, motor and nervous system of an individual and an 'animal' is called maturation. Individual of different species undergo different sequential patterns of development and maturation. It has been observed that unless an individual attends a particular level of maturation, he cannot learn a particular skill or learning. Different learning's require different levels of maturation. Acquisition of simple motor skills is possible in early infancy. But complex skills like writing and problem solving require a developed brain.

Here, in this context the important aspect is 'critical period' for learning. It has been observed that if a particular behavior or skill has not been learnt, a particular stage of child's maturational development, it becomes difficult for him to master it later on. This particular development stage is called the 'critical period' for that particular learning.

According to Harlow (1962), he studied on monkeys regarding critical period of particular learning. He raised some monkeys in isolation, without letting them to mix or play with other monkeys. He analyzed that, if the isolation is up to 90 days, the resultant abnormal social and sexual behavior is short-lived. But if isolation is more than that period, the abnormality persists throughout life. Thus, he came to conclusion that the first 90 days is the critical period for learning of social and sexual behavior in monkeys.

13. Learning is dependent on nervous system: Learning is also dependant on nervous system and brain. It has been found that the animals with more complex nervous system learn faster and acquire complex skills than those with simpler nervous systems. An environmentalist reared a chimpanzee just like a baby soon after its birth. He also gave it special training whenever necessary. As a result of this, she learnt to perform simpler acts like dusting, washing dishes and painting, etc. But she could not talk. That is because of the deficiency in the language or speech at the center of her brain. Thus limitations of the brain is an important factor in the learning ability of a child or an animal. For human learning, the growth of cerebral cortex plays a very important role. Growth of learning ability during the childhood and the adolescence is directly related to maturation of the cerebral cortex. The decline of learning ability in old age is probably due to the decay of that tissue of this part of the brain.

Lashly conducted a study on white rats. His three important things about learning and the brain are: the first is that learning is related to the amount of cortical tissue available inside the brain of the subject. The grater the amount of cortical tissues, the quicker will be learning. He proved this by taking away various percentages of cortical tissues from the brains of rats and then making them learn the maze. The second conclusion is that learning is related to the location of specific cortical tissues in the brain of the subject. He proved that the removal of specified cortical tissues led to the loss of sensitivity to visual details, removing another, to the loss of sensitivity to different odors and so on. Thus there are functions specialization inside the brain.

If the subject's brain lacks a particular center, say speech center, he cannot learn that ability. He also found that if a particular center in a brain of the subject, relating to some particular ability, is destroyed, then it results only in temporary loss of that ability. Gradually other parts of the cerebral cortex take up the functions of the destroyed center. Hence the lost ability of the subject reappears from this; he propounded his theory of mass action, which states that cerebrum functions as a mass, i.e. as a whole not as isolated specialized centers.

14. Learning is self-acting process: Learning is also a self-active process. Learning involves the subject. If a child has to learn he has to be involved in the process of learning. He has to participate in his experiences and has to learn from them. There cannot be any learning without the involvement of himself. To learn, a child or a subject has not only to involve his senses but he has also to use the higher centers of his brain, which will impart pattern, meaning and significance to his sensory inputs.

CHARACTERISTICS OF LEARNING

Learning is a process that provides impetus for a new behavior or through interaction with the environment brings change in the earlier behavior. But the change in behavior is not due to medicines. Learning brings a permanent change in behavior. Hence, the changes in behavior caused by regular exercise, games, habitual walks, taking drugs are not permanent. They may change the behavior for time being but not at all life-long or permanent manner. Change in the intensity of emotion may also bring change in behavior. So it is well to conclude that human behavior is the central theme of learning process. Behavior includes biopsychosocial activities in toto.

According to Mc Caw the characteristics of learning includes:

1. Learning is a continuous modification of behavior. The modification is relatively permanent as because the possibility of having the earlier form of behavior is very less. It is also a continuous process in the sense that the modification is continuous throughout in life.
2. Learning is pervasive. It relates to all aspects of human life.
3. Learning involves the whole person-social, emotional, psychological, economical and intellectual. There cannot be any learning without the involvement of the whole self of the learner.
4. Learning is a developmental process. A subject not only learns, he also simultaneously develops or improves his behavior. Whatever he learns makes him to have improved responses to his environment.
5. Learning is often a change in the organization of behavior.
6. Learning is responsive to incentives, positive incentives such as reward to help the learner learn quickly. Negative incentives such as punishment help to unlearn what has been learnt. But it has been proved that positive incentives are more effective in achieving their objective than the negative ones.
7. Learning is always goal directed. The goal generally appears as the solution of a certain problem, presented by the

environment of the learner. It might be the problem of passing the examination as in the problem of finding food stored at the end of the maze, as in the case of rat ready to learn the map of the maze.

8. Learning is the positive correlation with interest. Interest makes learning easier.
9. Learning depends upon maturational readiness and also on motivation.

Learning Process

Learning is a life long process. It is from cradle to grave. It begins with life and ends with life. It involves constant change, adjustment and development. It implies acquisition of knowledge and skills on the one hand, modification of behavior on the other. It is measured in terms of improvement of behavior. Learning facilitates the modification of behavior in new situations.

The process of learning is that by virtue of which the individual develops necessary skills and abilities so as to benefit himself from the past experiences. Learning process is that where a motivated individual succeed in a situation which he perceives as leading to a goal.

Factors Influencing Learning

Learning is a life long process. This depends upon a number of factors. They are classified as personal and environmental factors. Personal factors:

1. The internal condition of the learner such as capacity, motivation, age, sex difference, experience, etc.
2. Nature of the subject to be learnt (e.g. range of learning, complexity or simplicity of learning materials, etc.)
3. Methods of learning (e.g. memorization, analysis, drilling, recitation, etc.)

Environmental: These include

1. *Age:* Children do more fare than adults. It is a general belief that learning ability decreases with increase in age. The new research in learning process showed that there is a fixed and definite age when learning ability of the child is maximum. Apart from this there is also a fixed age for better learning of literature, mathematics, and science. There is a relationship

between age factor and learning. The learning ability of new subjects goes on increasing till the age of 10 years. Then it remains constant till age of 20 years and after that it goes on diminishing and again becomes stable at the age of fifty years.

2. *Role of gender in learning:* The new research in gender differences of learning shows the following findings.
   i. Difference in gender does not cause any difference in their intelligence.
   ii. While girls show more proficiency in literature, debate, song, etc. the boys show more ability in social science, science and mathematics, etc.
   iii. Girls are more emotional, sociable and jealous. Boys are more influential, high minded and independent minded and self confident.
   iv. Girls have greater pronouncing ability, better memory and sounder sensitiveness. On the other hand, boys show good result in numerology.
   v. Girls are interested in service, choice, home science, and literature, where as boys show interest in scientific technological and ideological fields.
3. *Role of mental stability in learning*: Effective learning and teaching depends fully upon a factor that is known as attention. Attention is the key for learning process. The learner should come in contact with the learning situation practically. He should attend by himself. Indirect participation yields very poor result.

   For example: If the students are told that they will be examined after 2 days of the learning, then they will take the situation more serious and also they are more attentive than testing after a fortnight. As result, learning outcome will be more effective and heightens the memory.
4. *Role of past experience in learning:* The present learning depends upon the learned past material. When a child fails in reading, writing or doing sums in classroom, it should be noted that he had a defective learning before hand, past learning enfuels present learning and at present learning smoothens the future learning process.
5. *Role of family background and socio-economic status in learning:* Urban and rural atmosphere contributes for learning. The

difference lies in their availability of stimulations. There are facilities such as libraries, magazines, periodicals, books, school, museum, TV and social networks. These stimulants tends to increase learning ability in children. Socio-economic status of students also a factor in learning. A child reared up in a luxurious environment is bound to be different from a child brought up in a poverty stricken family. The social customs and tradition, casteism, feeling of success and failure, financial status also contributes for learning.

6. *Role of experience of success and failure in learning:* A feeling of inferiority and hopelessness is marked in failure students. Usually children having high hopes become successful in life. So success and failure have their respective impacts on the learning process.
7. *Role of knowledge of promotion in learning:* Knowledge of promotion stimulates the learner and heightens his attention. The research shows that learning is impossible unless the learner knows the result of his last learning. So knowledge of result brings success in a new learning.
8. *Role of meaningfulness of subject matter in learning:* The meaningful materials are remembered better than the meaningless materials. Meaningful materials denotes those materials about which we have some previous experience.
9. *Role of complexity of material in learning:* Primarily, learning should start from simple and easy subject. Later complexity can be introduced. So, teaching-learning process should be from simple to complex. If child is presented complex subject at the beginning, he may show low proficiency and many chances are for his failure. He feels bored and neglects his studies and tries to get rid off it.
10. *Speed of learning materials:* According to Ebbinghaus, his study findings shows that a long list of words take a longer time to memorize than a short list. But it has also been proved that a bigger topic is remembered better and sooner than the shorter topic.
11. *Role of re-memorization in learning:* Re-memorization has a strong effect on learning and memorization, rememorization is also described as mental evaluation of learnt materials. Learning the material again is known as learning by closing the book. The mechanism of this process works as follows:

a. Re-memorization is a conscious effort and not only a bird's eye view, has it become fruitful.
b. The learner can measure his memorization by this process. So he can be aware of his limitations and weakness in learning. Learner knows what he failed to remember and invents methods to remember them again.
c. Re-memorization creates self-confidence in the learner.

12. *Role of over-learning:* Over learning brings good result. The topic which is remembered after the recitation of two or more times can be remembered better than after five more times. This helps the learner to produce the material more perfectly. Relearning is required to memorize but over learning makes the goal of learning felt. Drilling brings out the correct response but of the learner but over learning confirms it.
13. *Role of time lapse between learning situations:* Learning the material of the subject is to be divided in parts and learned by day wise, week wise and month wise. This enhances the speed and memorization of the topic under study.
14. *Difference between the whole method and part method:* In past, part method was popular but a now-a-days the whole method is practiced. In part method a longer topic is learnt in parts which makes the learning mechanical and the learner goes far from the root or basic point of the subject. Correlation could not be established among the various points of method. They were regarded by the learner as the different topic not as the points of view of only one topic. On the other hand, efficiency increased in whole learning and learning was still more effective. And if at all a vast subject is to be divided it should be done in such a manner as so the divisions are inter-related and interdependent. In whole method of learning, stress is laid upon the totality of the view point. The success of whole method depends upon the past experience of the learner, his temperament and complexity of material. If the subject matter is easy, interdependent, understandable and smooth it is learnt effectively.
15. *Recitation in learning:* Recitation at the time of reading a material makes learning more effective. Reading and recitation should go hand in hand.
16. *Use of audio-visual aids in learning:* Use of effective and appropriate audio-visual aids helps in learning efficiency. It needs a lot of preparation.

17. *Environmental factors:* The concept of critical period brings out the importance of environmental stimulation for learning. The human behavior is the response to the demand made by the environment. One can learn if there are opportunities and facilities in the environment to learn. It is found from research that, children from slums or orphanages, criminal background parents are of lesser caliber than children from stimulating environment. If the environment is deficient and there by is incapable to stimulate the child's inherent capabilities for learning. Thus his learning will be retarded and vice versa.

Theories of Learning

Learning theory has two purposes. One is that it gives detailed information about human behavior, supplies material for further research, brings to surface new facts and search of ultimate truth. Secondly a theory explains the relationship between different factors and interaction among them and its outcome.

Learning theories are divided into the following categories:

1. Association theories of learning
2. Cognitive theories of learning
3. Cybernetic theories of learning.

Association Theories of Learning

Association theories emphasizes the significance of "Association" or "Bond", which exists between stimulus and response. This theory claims that doing or undoing of a response-pattern is intimately related to the strength or weakness of this "connection". When the stimulus is repeated again and again there develops an association between the stimulus and the response, but when the stimulus is withdrawn and its frequency of occurrence is decreased the result out bond between the two gets weakened. The great theorists of this association are Thorndike's, Pavlov's, Guthrie and skinner, etc.

Trial and Error Learning: Edward L Thorndike (1874–1949) proposed laws of learning of voluntary responses. The theory states that at the beginning of learning a task, it takes time to complete the task and many errors are committed in the course of learning. But as number of trials increase, the errors will be reduced. *For example:* Learning to ride a bicycle, the beginner rider crumbles and gets hurt. As he practices daily, the task become easy.

Thorndike conducted an experiment on cat. He made a 'puzzle box'. He kept a hungry cat in a cage and a piece of meat just out side of the cage. He kept a lever within the cage and pressing of it can open the door of cage. In the beginning cat made many efforts by attacking on the bars of the cage with paw and bites. But it has failed. However, by chance the lever was pressed and cat came out of cage. In another chance cat made attempt but shortly came out. As the trials continuous, cat learnt to open the cage and escaped out quickly in later stages of learning.

From the above experiment, he formulated laws of learning:

1. Law of exercise
2. Law of readiness
3. Law of effect.

Law of Exercise

It states that if a task is repeated many times, it will be learnt. *For example:* Words can be read again and again by mnemonics. Thus repetition makes the response more and stronger with practice, i.e. practice makes the man perfect.

Law of Readiness

Learning requires readiness or preparedness on the part of the learner. Thorndike comments "when any conduction unit is in readiness to conduct, for it to do so is satisfying; when any conduction units is not in readiness to conduct, for it to conduct is annoying, when any conduction unit is in readiness to conduct, for it not to do is annoying". This explains that readiness is closely associated with the condition of the individual especially that of nervous system. Learning will take place when only the learner is "ready". If the learner is not ready physically and mentally, the experiences would be annoying, dissatisfying and displeasing.

Law of Effect

This law is also known as "law of satisfaction and annoyance" or "reward and punishment". Thorndike observed that "when a modifiable connection between a situation and a response is made and is accompanied or followed by a satisfying state of affairs, that connection strength is increased, when made or accompanied or followed by an annoying state of affairs; its strength is decreased.

In the beginning, most activities of the child are accompanied either by bodily pain or pleasure. Pleasure makes the child repeat the activity, dissatisfaction causes avoidance. Play is a pleasurable activity, it is part and parcel of the child's instinctive behavior. Any situation which irritates during play, may frustrate the child and lead to an annoying state. Satisfaction brings success; success leads to further accomplishment. It builds confidence, keeps the interest in the activity alive.

Sub Laws of Learning

Law of contiguity: Law of contiguity states that situation which occur together either simultaneously or in close succession tend toward reviving one another.

For example: The Taj Mahal denotes use of Agra, Shahjan, Mumtaz Mahal, the river Yamuna, etc. because of their association.

Law of multiple response to the same external situation: This law is also known as concomitant or attendant learning. It states that the individual makes several responses and not one to the same situation or the external stimulus. A chance word or observation sets off train thoughts which run for a long time. Some external stimulus seems to be necessary in the beginning but once a series of reactions starts, it provides its own stimulus for continuance of the further internal or external activity, i.e. one reaction leads to a number of further reaction in sequence. Then multiple responses to a single stimulus. In this process, the desirable responses may be selected and practiced and the undesirable ones eliminated. The higher the animal's status in the hierarchy of the evolutionary scale, the greater the number and the variety of responses. This shows the variability of human behavior.

For example: during an athletic class, the learner not only learns the activity pattern but also how he explains the procedures, teaches what techniques, what peculiar word or sentences he uses to make teaching, more effective. All these factors ultimately decide whether the learner would give response partially or wholly.

Law of mental set: Learning is guided by total attitude or set of the organism. Learner knows his own aspiration.

Laws of partial activity: The response elicited by a particular stimulus may not be fully applicable for the stimulus. It may be applicable for a part of it.

For example: a person meets another person, and responds in a particular way. This response is aroused by noticing the face of the stimulus person. His dresses and behavior get unnoticed and have a no part to play in the ground of such a response. So here the response is partial.

Principle of analogy: This is also called as "from known to unknown". Here, the learner assimilates and compares the new situation to a previously learned and gives a response by analogy.

Principle of associative shifting: Stimulating situations change, but the response remains unchanged, it is called associative shifting.

For example: a dog can be trained to stand up by showing piece of meat. Then it can stand up only by giving orders. By associative shifting means get any response of which a learner is capable associated with any situation to which he is sensitive. It is also called "substituting a conditioned stimulus or an unconditioned one".

CLASSICAL CONDITIONING THEORY

Classical conditioning theory was postulated by a Soviet Russian Psychologist Ivan Pavlov and won Nobel Prize in 1904 for his outstanding contribution on the psychology of digestion.

Conditioning learning takes place at a lower level. It is nothing but the "establishment of connection between a stimulus and a response which have no natural connection between them".

Pavlov demonstrated that a dog salivates when food is put into its mouth. This reflex of salivation is physiological and natural. But the dog can be made to salivate to any other neutral stimulus, say the sound of the bell, for a few times the natural stimulus (food) is presented to the dog with the neutral stimulus (i.e. sound of the bell). This salivation, the sound of bell is unnatural and learned. Pavlov named the natural stimulus for salivation, i.e. food, was called by him as unconditioned stimulus (US). The natural responses to it, i.e. salivation while eating was called unconditioned response (UR). The experimental stimulus which was neutral before experiment, but to which response in conditioned (i.e. connected) during experiment is called conditioned stimulus (CS). Here it is sound of the bell. The learned response (i.e. salivation) to the otherwise neutral stimulus (i.e. sound of the bell) is called conditioned response (CR).

Pavlov experimented on dogs. He paired food and bell a few times. It was found that after a few pairing, the dog salivates even when only bell is sounded and food is not presented. This salivation is nothing but a conditioned (i.e. learned) response to neutral stimulus, i.e. bell. Thus, classical conditioning is a process in which a neutral stimulus by pairing with a natural stimulus, acquires all the characteristics of neutral stimulus.

I stage			
	Food	Salivation	
	Bell	No salivation	
II stage			
	Bell	Food	Salivation
III stage			
	Bell	Salivation	

Fig. 3.3: Pavlov's experiment design (Reference: Psychology Munn and Munn)

Cognitive theory

JB Watson and Edwin R Guthrie are the exponents of theory of conditioning without reinforcement. According to them contiguity occurrence at the same time is enough to establish a bond or connection between stimulus and a response. They also believe that all stimulus response connections learnt by man have their corresponding reflections on human nervous system.

Behaviorist Theory of Learning

Behaviorism started in America with the publication of Watson's book (1878–1959) 'Psychology'. According to Watson, behavior is a response to stimulus. It is a stimulus response S-R connections, e.g. sneezing to irritation in nose. These are simple unconditioned reflexes or simple S-R unit. But new stimulus and response reactions are also learnt by us by process of conditioning. Our habits and other complex behaviors are the results of the chains or series of such conditioned reflexes. Learning is the change of behavior arising out of the new S-R connections or reflexes.

Watson proposed that when a stimulus and a response occur at the same time in contiguity, connection between them is established. The strength of connection between a stimulus and a response depends upon the frequency of S-R repetitions. This is known as Watson's law of frequency. The more frequently a response had been connected to a stimulus in the past, the more it is likely that we will give that response to that stimulus in future. Another law is called law of recency. The more recently we have given a response to a stimulus in future.

Theory of Continuous Conditioning or Simultaneous Conditioning

This theory is developed by Edwin R Guthrie (1886–1959) of the Washington University was a neobehaviorist. The learning theory of Guthrie stresses that the organism responds to various stimuli by contraction of muscles and secretion of glands. There specific responses are called movements by Guthrie. An act is a series of movements by associated together by the contiguity of time. *For example:* the act of dancing consists of various separate movements of muscles and senses.

Simultaneous conditioning means association between stimulus and response by contiguity of time. If a particular type of stimulus elicit a particular response. Thus in nutshell, Guthrie advocates that what is learnt is only a bond between the stimulus and the response of the organism is the from of glandular i.e. secretions of muscular contractions and expansions.

Instrumental or Operant Conditioning

Operant conditioning theory was proposed by BF Skinner, a Harvard psychologist. He developed as "technology" of behavior. He opines that all of us are controlled by our physical surroundings as well as by other people. Such control may be subtle, but it is always present. The fundamental mechanism of control is reinforcement. We learn to do the thing that either reward or permit us to avoid pain. In short, reinforcement determines our behavior.

Type of Behavior and Conditioning

Respondent Behavior and Type-S Conditioning

Responses that are "elicited" by known stimuli are called as respondent. Pupillary construction to light, salivation at sight of food and other reflex actions fell under this category. Skinner calls such conditioning of respondent of 'Type-S' conditioning.

Operant Behavior and Type-R Conditioning

Responses 'emitted' by the subject rather than being elicited by the stimulus. This is active control of the organism and operates on the environment. Hence, it is known as operant behavior. Skinner believes that when any operant behavior of the subject is followed by a reward, then there will be more likelihood of that behavior to occur in future. In other words that behavior will be learnt for that situation. He named this conditioning as 'Type-R' conditioning.

Concept of Reinforcement

BF Skinner introduced the concept of reinforcement. It means to strengthen and he defined it is anything that, when following a response, causes that response to be more likely to happen again. Reinforcers are primary and secondary in nature. Primary reinforcer satisfies the basic need of organisms like food, liquid (thirst drive). Infants, children and animals can be easily reinforced by using primary reinforcers.

A secondary reinforcer is the one gets its properties from primary reinforcers in the past. *For example:* If a person praises a puppy while petting him (sense of touch, primary reinforcer), the praise makes the puppy squirm with delight.

Positive and Negative Reinforcement

Positive Reinforcement: It occurs when a stimulus presented following an operant response strengthens the probability of occurrence of that response food, water, sexual contact, etc. are positive reinforcers for the individual's deprived of those items.

Negative Reinforcement: It is the reinforcement of a response by the removal, escape from, or avoidance of an unpleasant stimulus. *For example:* Lying of the behavior results in avoiding an unpleasant stimulus (the scolding). Another example is punishment always descreases the likelihood of a behavior happening again. Punishment weakens responses, whereas reinforcement strengthens responses.

Cognitive Theories of Learning

The proponents of cognitive theories are Kohler, Tolman, Lewin, Comb and Rogers, etc. who are the opinion that the individual in the process going through novel experiences discovers "meaningful relationship in order to solve problems". Cognitive theorists firmly believe that the ultimate control of behavior lies within the cognitive structure of a person. Cognition is "knowing" the situation fully and bearing its impression in one's mind. The 'inner' self does the activity again before the impulse travels outward to involve musculature. Inner activity is a prerequisite of any outer experience.

Gestalt Theories of Learning And Theory of Insinght

The word 'Gestalt' is a German word which means "pattern" or "Shape" or "configuration". The Gestalt psychologists like Max Wertheimer, Wolfgang Kohler, Jurt KoffKa, etc. believe that our perception of the world is in terms of patterns, shapes, forms or configurations which are meaningful wholes. These wholes are different and more than the parts they are composed of. According to them, learning is a secondary and derivative phenomenon, the starting point of their treatment of learning is the belief that the laws of organization perception is equally applicable to learning situation also, since the laws of organization structure the perceptions of events and information they also equally determine what is stored in our memory after such perception and also what is recalled.

Insight Theory of Learning

It is actually propounded by Thorndike. The end result of his experiments on animals yielded that problems are solved by trail and error method. Actually man and higher animals like primates solve their problem by insight, i.e. by understanding.

Characteristics of Insightful Learning

1. Insightful learning is sudden; Unlike conditioning is not progressive.

2. There is feeling of understanding. The learner gets an understanding, i.e. insight into the different relations between the elements in the problem situation.
3. It is better retained than 'trial and error' learning. Since the learner learns the material with understanding, the traces are resistant to change.
4. It is transferred heavily into similar new situation.

Educational Implications of Insightful Theory

Educational psychologists view the insight theory is of more importance than other theories. These are:

1. Proceeding from Whole to the Part: According to Gestalt theory learning process should proceed from whole of the subject matter to various parts of it. By teaching the whole topic, a complete idea is captured in mind.

For example: at the time of teaching intra venous injection, the teacher should start from the related anatomy and physiology of nervous system then to the concerned part.

2. Creation of Motivation: Creation is an art and science. So the teacher has the duty to motivate the students to study. Motivator can only help into action of learning.

3. Emphasis on Understanding: Trial and error, mechanical repetition and learning by rote is not considered a very effective use in higher studies. More complex studies can be solved by insightful learning. Here there is no fear of time and energy.

Insightful learning is not proved fruitful in case of learners having a low intelligence and slow learners. They can learn effectively by trail and error. Apart from the although some difficult problems can be solved by insight, the more difficult and critical problems cannot be solved by mere is insight and general cognition.

Observational Learning

Observational learning is the learning of new behavior though the act of observation of a model. This learning theory was proposed by Bandura in 1961. The experiment on children in observational learning yield that learning can take place without actual performance. Observational learning includes four elements. Attention, memory, imitation and motivation are the principle components of observational learning.

Machine Learning

Traditionally, it is thought that learning takes place only in animals, but now computers are also can modify their own behaviors as a result of experiences. This is known as machine learning. It is nothing but artificial intelligence concerned with the design and development of algorithms and techniques that allow computers to "learn". It involves two types of learning. Inductive and deductive. Inductive machine learning methods extract rules and patterns out of massive data sets. The major function of machine learning is to extract information from data automatically by computational and statistical methods. It is closely related to data mining and statistics and theoretical computer science.

Rote Learning

This learning is by repetition. It avoids understanding the inner complexities and inferences of the subject and only focuses on memorizing the material so that it can be recalled by the learner exactly the way it was read or heard.

Informal Learning

Informal learning is an unorganized and learning at home and at work. Informal learning is what happens when knowledge has not been externalized or captured and exists only inside someone's head. To get at the knowledge, you have to meet and talk to him. Examples of informal learning transfer include instant messaging, a spontaneous meeting on computer net, a chat-room in real time, etc.

Formal learning

Learning in a place within student-teacher relationship, specialized courses as a system. It takes place in schools and colleges.

Learning Organization

The learning organization is one that learns continuously and transforms itself. Learning takes place in individuals, teams, the organization and even the communities with which the organization interacts. Learning is a continuous, strategically used process integrated with and running parallel to, work. Learning results in changes in knowledge, beliefs and behaviors. Learning also enhances organizational capacity for innovation and growth. The learning organization has embedded system to capture and share learning.

MEMORY

We learn many things daily. What we learnt past is used now. It is because the memory of learning and experiences are retained in mind. Retentation is also a part of memory.

Memory is the process of remembering objects of past experience. It is a representative process. It involves retention and sense of recall of reproduction.

Meaning of Memory

Memory is a special ability of mind through which learning can be retained and reproduced if and when required. It has a three fold function of mind rather than a power but involves learning, retaining and remembering.

Nature of Memory

Nature of memory may be discussed under three parts:

1. *Learning:* This is the first step where individual needs to drive sense experience of the environment in order to register its impression called learning. It consists of sensing and perceiving the object of experience in mind.
2. *Retaining/Storage:* Retaining/storage is learning experience received is being tried to retain in mind in the form of image. After there is always an effort to keep its image in mind intact in the subconscious level. This retaining mostly inherited by birth.
3. *Remembering/ Retrieval:* This is the third step where we try to reproduce the past image in the present in its original form called remembering. It is an act of exchanged reproduction of what was retained in mind in the past. This mental revival or remembering may again take the form of recall and recognition. Recall is the independent recollection of the past

where as recognition is the verification of the given experience on the basis of image of the past.

From above points, we can say that memory is a part of mental act of retaining and reviving of the past learning and experience. It involves three fold mental functions of learning, retaining and remembering.

Definitions

The concept of memory has been defined by the theorists as follows:

- James S Ross—"A memory is a new experience determined by the dispositions laid down by a previous experience, the relation between the two being clearly apprehended.
- Woodworth—"Memory consists of learning, retaining and remembering what has previously been learned".
- Baddeley (2003)—Memory is an active system that receives information from the senses, organizes and alters it as it stores it away and then receives the information from storage.
- Eyesenck defined as memory is the ability of the organism to store information from earlier learning processes and reproduce that information in answer to specific stimuli.

Characteristics/Functions of Memory

The nature and function of memory are:

1. Memory depends on the power of retaining which is inherited by birth.
2. Memorizing is a mechanical activity that lacks the creativity of mind.
3. It is an exact and unchanged reproduction of the past experiences in mind.
4. Unconscious mind plays an important role in exercise of one's memory.
5. Repetition makes memory image more durable and lasting.
6. Memory needs direct experience of senses, in the absence of which the question of memory does not arise.
7. Memory needs intellectual ability and better power of mental organization of individual.

Factors Influencing Memory

The following factors determine the process of memory:

1. Acquisition of Experience: Acquisition of experience or learning is a process of forming association among ideas in the mind. Physiopsychologically it consists informing connections between neurons. Memory also includes learning. If the subject is learnt well, it will be reproduced very well, in the absence of it, there will be not be any true function of memory. The efficient the learning, the better is the reproduction.

2. Retention: The learnt material leaves a mark on brain in the form of structural modification, i.e. physiological disposition. Remembering or recall depends on retention.

3. Recall/Reproduction: It is bringing the information from subconscious level to the consciousness.

For example: a learnt chapter can be revived now. This is known as recall or reproduction.

4. Recognition: This is the feeling of familiarity which accompanies the revival of the past.

For example: I see an old friend of mine, I recognize him as one of my classmates. This sort of mental process is recognition which is an import function of memory. Here, sense perception plays a vital role, i.e. individual must have the familiarity.

Conditions of Good Memory

Memory differs from individual to individual. It mainly has genetic composition. However, retention also varies with one's age, health condition, etc. To retain good retention, one has to follow the following methods:

1. Repetition/over learning
2. Self-recitation
3. The method of distribution or spaced practice
4. Adoption of whole part methods of practice
5. Association and meaningfulness
6. Imagery
7. Organization
8. The motivation
9. Positive attitude and variance, etc.

Types of Memory

The learnt material cannot be stored for life long. On the basis of duration of retention of material, it is divided in to the following types:

1. Sensory memory
2. Short-term memory (STM)
3. Long-term memory (LTM).

1. Sensory Memory: In sensory memory, memory traces are retained at sense organs for a second of time. Further memory traces fade away and the subject matter is forgotten.

2. Short-term Memory (STM): In short-term memory, the memory system in which information is held for very brief periods of time while being used. It may range from few seconds to few minutes. In this memory, the learnt material is retained in the brain in the form of circular neural connection which can be broken easily by extrinsic factors. The material is retained as long on the bioelectric channel keep as circulating in the neural circuit. As the neural circuit is broken, material is forgotten.

For example: Dialing a telephone number and afterwards forgetting.

3. Long-term Memory (LTM): In LTM, the system into which all the information is placed to be kept more or less permanently. It is unlimited in capacity.

The material is retained for many minutes, hours, days, months, years, and decades.

For example: elder people do remember their preschool moments. Long-term memory depends on the law of association. The more the learned material is associated with other ideas in the mind, the greater is the permanency.

4. Active and Passive Memory: Passive or spontaneous memory, is that type of memory, where past learnt experiences/skills are recalled without any effort of the will.

For example: river Ganges remembers a lot, like the purity of water, the history and mythology. But when we remember past learnt experiences by one effort of the will, it is known as achieve memory or recollection.

For example: Remembering a childhood friend by effort and force.

5. Personal or Impersonal Memory: Memory is also personal in nature. Some individuals have good memory about their personal experiences and others for impersonal experiences as well. The former consists of personal past experiences and the later impersonal experiences.

For example: I cannot forget the day, when I received my award at Delhi, and took pride in thinking myself the same. This is personal memory, but when I recall my experience in a letter to my friend, it becomes an impersonal memory.

6. Rote Memory and Logical Memory: Rote memory depends on the mechanical repetition of the material and logical memory involves proper reasoning, understanding and logical organization of facts. It also involves more psychological, because it involves self-consciousness. Attitudes, inner urges and interest of the learner:

Models/Theories of Memory

To explain the mechanism of memory, researchers put forth models and theories. The most influential theories regarding memory are:

i. Information processing model
ii. Neuro-cognitive theory.

1. Information-Processing Model (IPM): Information processing model is an approach that focuses on the way information is processed or handled through encoding, storage and retrieval stages of memory. It assumes that how long a memory will be remembered depends on the stage of memory in which it is stored. According to information processing model, it looks at how thought processes like memory work, uses as its model for human thought the way that computer functions. Data are encoded in brain as like computer can understand and use. The computer stores that information on a memory disk and then the data are retrieved out of storage as needed. These theorists primly proposed three stages of memory systems as sensory memory, short-term memory and long term memory.

Flow chart 3.1: Information processing model

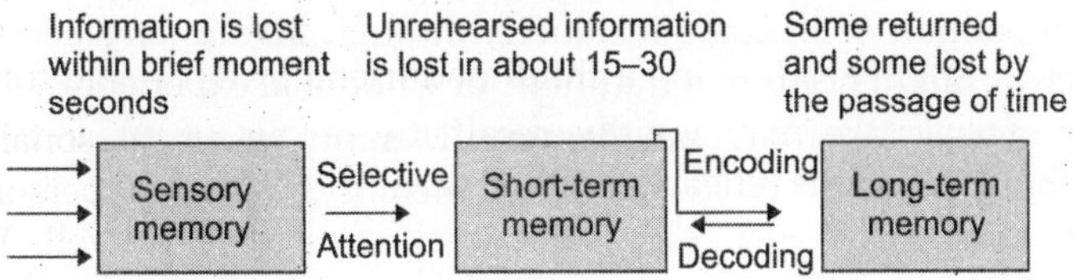

Process of Memory

The Neurocognitive Theory of Memory

The current research in neurocognition of memory involve the plotting of functions on the topography of the brain, the routing of memory traces and the identification of the neural changes in the brain associated with memory formation and change. In brain, three sites seems to be directly involved in memory system. These sites are the cortex of the brain thought to be involved in higher-order cognition such as thinking, problem solving and remembering: the cerebellum at the base of the brain involved in the regulation of motor functions and motor memory; and the hippocampus is believed to process new information and route it to parts of the cortex for permanent storage. The newer research findings suggest two types of memories, procedural and declarative memory are associated with these major structures. Procedural memory deals with motor skills where as declarative memory consists of information and knowledge of the world, such as the name of a favorite friend, meaning of words and a vast information is stored in the cerebral cortex.

Sensory information is routed in the cortex soon after it is experienced. There temporary links are formed among neurons and persist only briefly; but long enough for uncomplicated actions to take place, such as remembering a telephone number till you dial. In order for these impressions to become permanent a process called long-term potentiation (LTP) occurs. This is the tendency of nerve cells that have been exposed to a rapidly repeated stimulus to enhance their response tendencies for an extended period of time. It occurs at hippocampus synapse. Actually, the dendrites stimulated, which facilitates long-term memories. Long term declarative memories are thought to begin as the cerebral cortex sends information to the hippocampus, a process that strengthens the memory by rapidly and repeatedly exciting the neural circuit in the cortex. The strengthening of long term memory may be achieved through voluntary actions, such as repetition or in some instances, through involuntary actions, such as might occur in a traumatic or emotional experience.

For example: we may vividly recall the details of an accident without conscious rehearsal of the event.

Methods of Memorizing: Good memory or memorization is an essential for any learner. Three factors contribute for memorization:

i. Proper encoding and storing of information
ii. Retaining
iii. Quick, prompt and correct retrieval of the information. Proper coding and storing of information can be done by use of organization, mental imagery. Retention of material can be achieved by repetition, recitation and spaced practice. Similarly, better retrieval can be effected by meaningful learning, organization, etc.

Repetition and Over-learning: To retain the skills and performance, repetition is must. Even after a mastery in any subject, it is advantageous to repeat it again. This over learning prevents the memory traces from fading out. The retention of skills like driving, cycling, swimming, etc. even after long disuse is because of the fact that they were repeated many more times even after their mastery. The proverb practice makes a man prefect suits for over learning.

Self-Recitation: Self-recitation is recalling the study material during practice or study. It increases the retention of the study material studied. Here, learner reads the study material, then asks questions about the material by himself. Then he studies the same material to clear his points which were doubtful at first. In self-recitation the individual is actively involved in learning process. Active involvement results in better retention and greater concentration and higher interest. All these contribute for better retention of study material in mind.

Spaced Practice: Spaced practice is the method by which the material is learnt with intervals over a period of days and months called spaced practice. According to CI Hovland's research conducted on type of practice, he made one group of subjects to learn unrelated syllables continuously while the other group learnt it with rest period in between. To keep constant the factors like the time taken for learning, the rate of exposure, etc. memory drum was used. The findings showed that the group following the continuous practice method required on an average more number of repetitions of the list, than the other groups.

Meaningfulness or Associations: The term meaningfulness is used to refer to the associations evoked by a material or an information, that is being learned. The greater the associations evoked by a material, the better will be its retention.

Forgetting: Learning includes forgetting. It is the failure to retain what has been learnt. According to Freudian theory, forgetting is the defense mechanism of mind. It helps the conscious mind to defend itself from the unpleasant and painful experiences that might cause anxiety and disturbances. Forgetting pushes them back to the region of unconscious called repression. Forgetting is therefore, a voluntary and active effort of on individual. It is deeply rooted in one's unconscious and hidden chamber of mind.

Definitions

Different psychologists define forgetting as follows:

Munn: Forgetting is the loss, permanent or temporary, of the ability to recall or recognize something learned earlier.

Drever: Forgetting means failure at any time to recall an experience, when attempting to do so, or to perform an action previously learned.

Forgetting is nothing but the failure of the individual to revive in consciousness an idea or group of ideas without the help of the original stimulus. Forgetting is the opposite of recall or remembering.

Causes: Usually we say that forgetting takes place with the passage of time. But, some other factors also contributes for it. Causes are at physical and psychological in origin. Physical factors are called fading and psychological factors are called blocking. These are:

1. *Head Injury:* Injury to cerebrum causes memory lapse. Physical diseases also causes loss of memory.
2. *Drug Addiction:* Drug abuse alters the mechanism of neurotransmitters in brain. This gives rise to temporary loss of memory.
3. *Old-Age and Intelligence:* Old age contributes for forgetting easily than youth. Similarly, intelligent people forget less than feeble minded people.
4. *Emotion Provoking Situation:* Emotion provoking situations accelerate forgetting.
5. *Fatigue:* Physical and psychological tiredness causes forgetting. Rest retains it.

6. *Break of Association:* Associative subject matter retains in the memory but unlinked matter yields to forgetting.
7. *Effacements of the Subconscious:* Effacements of the subconscious traces of past experience causes forgetting.
8. *Repression:* Painful experiences are repressed and tries to forgetfulness.
9. *Closer:* When learning continues, learner will be active but learner comes to a close or end, anxiety disappears and learner feel relief. It results in forgetting very easily.
10. *Retro-Active Inhibition:* When time lapse is more in learning different materials, it leads to forgetting.
11. *Want for Review:* After learning a subject a learner is required to review it by repetition. If he failed to do so what has been learnt fades away.

Types of Forgetting: Forgetting is classified into natural and morbid forgetting. In natural forgetting, forgetting occurs with the lapse of time in quite a normal way without any intention of forgetting on the part of the individual whereas in morbid or abnormal forgetting, one deliberately tries to forget the matter. According to Freud, it results from repression and is wishful as one happens to forget the thing which he does not wish to remember.

Theories of Forgetting: Actually, how the forgetting occurs still under research. Many theorists put forth their explanations. These are:

1. *Memory Trace Decay Theory:* This is a very old theory put forth for forgetting. According to this theory, physical changes in the brain, perhaps in a neuron or in the activity between neurons and disuse of traces of memory yields to decay, fading into nothing. This causes forgetting.
2. *Interference Theory*: According to this theory, forgetting results from interference between items of information stored in memory. Interference may be retroactive and proactive interference. In retroactive interference, information currently being learned interferes with information already present in memory.

   For example: learning a new computer program cause to forget the already learned material. In proactive interference, the previously learned information present in long-term memory interferes with information which we are learning at present.

   For example: Suppose you learned how to operate one TV, now you buy a new one, which requires different steps to operate. If you now make mistakes by trying to operate the new TV in the same way as you did the old, this constitutes proactive interference.

Improvement of Memory: Improvement of memory is not actually possible like improvement of muscles or body building. According to William Mc Dougall, memory can be improved by practice. But, William James views that one's native retentiveness is unchangeable. Practice may improve the power of retaining. Through special training, we can channelize the memory process for efficiency, but general memory power remains unchanged. From these views it appears that improvement of memory is not an easy task and person cannot convert bad memory into a good memory. However, some of the following favorable conditions can contribute to improve memory.

Flow chart 3.2: Process of memory

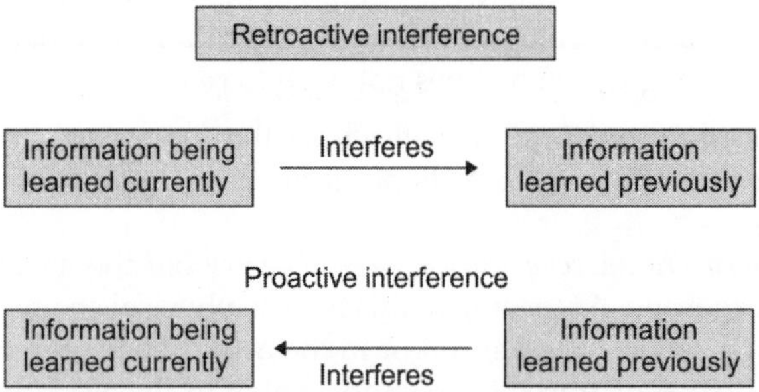

These are as follows:

1. *Desire to Learn:* An individual cannot learn unless he/she has desire to do so. Learning needs an active volition, a receptive mood and a momentary interest in the learning task before any success can be anticipated. Materials read, heard or seen without intention or mood are not remembered for long time. It shows that for keeping a memory a long time, it requires an urge to learn with intention.
2. *Motive:* Education is power. The learner should know the objective and output of learning. Aimless learning gives rise

to failure. The learner gets incentive to learn by the help of motive.

3. *Regular Practice:* Timely repetition of subject matter helps to keep the experiences fresh and active in mind. Since it revitalizes the image forgetting cannot influence memory.
4. *Use of Active Method:* Learning may be active or passive. Active learning is concerned by learning by doing. Following the active method, learning experiences remain active in mind for a long period.
5. *Rest and Leisure:* Regular rest and leisure in between study periods helps to overcome fatigue and boredom, this helps to revitalize the mind and body.
6. *Conscious Effort to Learn:* Conscious effort to learn invokes attention. This helps to keep the learned matter actively in mind.
7. *Proper Understanding:* Proper critical understanding of the material plays a vital role in memorization. Only mechanical method or blind imitation results in poor results.
8. *Learning though Experiments:* This is nothing but learning by doing. Pragmatic approach to learning helps the sense organs to be active and retention span will be more.
9. *Practice of Whole Method:* Whole method of learning makes impression permanent. It helps the learner to get a total picture of learning which is permanent.
10. *Practice of Rehearsal and Recitation:* Rehearsal and recitation are instrumental in memorizing as they afford an opportunity of self presentation and presentation through other senses. When we recite we use speech and hearing both besides the right through which the material is initially presented. Rehearsal gives a chance of self evaluation and confidence in learning.
11. *Use of Rhythm:* Rthymic materials help the learner to memorize the learning materials effectively.

Nursing Perceptives: Learning is from cradle to grave. Nurses must acclimatize the value of learning. They have to understand the importance of associative learning and role of reinforcement specially in the management of psychiatric clients. Nurses can imbibe the newer methods of memorization which helps them to teach the memory distorted clients. Theoretical knowledge of learning can be implemented in clinical areas.

THINKING

Man is unique in nature. Our abilities to think and speak made the world a beautiful living. The thoughts are transformed as language. Thinking has made a vivid transformation of this universe.

Thinking or cognition refers to the use of perceptions, mental combinations and internal representation of symbols, objects or concepts.

Thinking encompasses all of the mental activities associated with concept formation, problem solving, intellectual functioning, creativity, complex learning, memory, symbolic processing, imagery, etc.

Nature of Thinking

Thinking is a mental process which involves the psychomotor system of our body-receptors, connectors and effectors, that is, sense organs, nerves and muscles. The connectors play a vital role in thinking. These are the neural mechanisms in the brain. When, thinking process occurs, people express is varied forms, such as biting the nail tips, clinching their fists, etc.

Thinking is a motivated process. It is a purposive mental activity. It is a process of dealing with ideas or thoughts or concepts. A concept can be defined as the relationship between, or the properties shared by the objects or ideas in a given group. Concept is the result of our perceptual experiences.

For example: table. We see their common qualities and characteristics, relations and finally conclude about generalized notion. We come to generalization as a result of perceptual experience, our ability to compare the common qualities, to relate them to each other, to abstract and generalize. As the concepts develop, we think it is the true sense of the world.

Concepts are expressed is the form of words of language. Words represent the concepts.

For example: the word horse, represents the idea or concept of horse which stands for all types of horses. In other meaning, language helps in thinking.

Types of Thinking

Thinking can be mainly categorized as:

1. Concept formation
2. Problem solving and reasoning

3. Decision making
4. Controlled and free thinking
5. Creative thinking
6. Imagination and dreaming
7. Means and ends analysis
8. Convergent and divergent thinking

Concept Formation: Concept formation is the most used way to organize thinking by forming concept. A concept is the relation between the objects or ideas in a given group. We develop concepts in part by classifying objects according to their similarly to other objects and the classification may occur even when the similarities are very abstract. Further, we tend to classify objects and ideas that appear to be similar under our conceptual heading until a difference because apartment. The same objects may also share many different conceptual categories, all of which are based on the persons knowledge of the similarities and differences between objects.

For example: It is gray color more like white or more like black? Gray hair is judged to be more white hair than black hair because of our knowledge of aging. However, gray clouds are judged to be more like black clouds than white clouds, because our knowledge of storms. Because we have knowledge about the world and how it operates, we adjust our conceptual categories accordingly.

Problem Solving and Reasoning: Problem solving occurs when a goal must be reached by thinking and behaving in a certain ways. Here, the thought process is directed consciously towards the solution of a difficulty or a problem. Solution can achieved in relation to the reality of the situation. Dreaming and reasoning are also the ways so solve the problem but in unrealistic ways. According to Sherman-Reasoning is a processes of thinking during which the individual is aware of a problem; identifies it; evaluates it and decides upon a solution. It is also helpful not only to solve immediate problem but also to future programs.

Steps in Problem Solving Process: The steps in problem solving involves the following:

1. *Awareness of the Problem:* The individual becomes aware of the problems and tries to known in depth about the situation.
2. *Comprehension of the problem:* Here, the problem is defined and analyzed. It is isolated from other problems. The difficulties in solving the problems are clearly understood. Information and other resources are gathered on the various aspects of the problem.

3. *Formulation of plans of Action:* The problem is understood in all the ways and comprehended. Plan of action is processed.
4. *Evaluation:* Plans are evaluated by keeping in mind, the suitability of resources. We choose the plan that solves or seems to solve our problem best.
5. *Practice and Verification:* The chosen plan is made to practice to know the 'rightness' by conclusions.

Decision-making: It includes inductive reasoning. Before decision-making, making the decision frame is necessary. A decision frame is a conception of the acts, outcomes and contingencies associated with a particular choice. Here, the norms, habits and personal characteristics play an important role.

Creative Thinking: It includes both reasoning and imagination. Here, creativity is used to solve the problem. The best example of creative thinking is an artist paints a picture. The artist has a goal, even if the exact nature of the goal is not clear. But the artist has greater freedom in his thoughts and ideas than is involved in problem-solving activities.

Controlled and Free Thinking: In controlled thinking we regulate and control the process of thinking. We see our thoughts keep in close touch with reality and are directed towards the achievement of a specific goal. Reasoning, problem solving and creative thinking includes controlled thinking.

In free thinking, thought processes are allowed much greater freedom of action. No restrictions of reality in time and space. There is no desire on the part of the thinker to achieve a certain goal which is realistic. The process of imagination, daydreaming and dreaming are typical examples of free thinking.

Imagination and Dreaming: Imagination is the culmination of images. It is a mental activity in which we make use of images and go beyond it. When we are imaging, we loose contact with real perception. We only have the mental image of the object or situation and create something a new of our own. For example, missing from a grave accident. It this scenario, after a long time, we call back the images of the experience.

Daydreaming: It is nothing but dreaming during working hours. It is an idle imagination, like building castles in the air. In day dreams, impossible things become possible, our wishes which cannot be fulfilled in real life are fulfilled. For example, a poor daydreaming, about a millionaire.

Dreaming: Dreaming takes place when we are asleep. Dream are mental activities of lighter sleep. They emerge in response to some stimulus either internal or external. Dream ideas or thoughts are generally strange, bizarre and incongruous because in our sleep, we lose contact with reality.

Means and End Analysis: Newell and Simon developed a computer planning and strategy program called the general problem solver (GPS) on the basis of heuristic philosophy is known as means-end analysis. It uses intellectual skills and facts (declarative knowledge).

Convergent and Divergent Thinking: In convergent thinking, the person starts from a number of points but eventually he will converge on the same solution of problem. This involves the application of one's knowledge and rules of logic and leads to a single possible answer.

For example: a nurse want to know why the patient on bed number 8 is so confused.

Divergent Thinking: It is creating many possible solutions from a single idea. Here variety of thoughts are involved. It is used for finding a number of alternatives to fit in a given situation, e.g. decorating the room in a limited budget. Here, creativity is used as a tool.

Levels of Thinking: Thinking starts with sounds of speech, spoken language. It has phonemes syllables, morphemes, words, clauses and sentences.

Phonemes: It is the minimal unit of speech in a given language that makes a difference to the fluent speaker of that language.

Syllables: The syllable is the smallest unit of speech perception.

Morphemes: These are the smallest unit in meaning in speech perception.

Clauses: It consists of a verb and its associated nouns. adjectives and so on. Clauses are the major units of perceived meaning in speech.

For example: "where there is a will" is one clause and its continuation, there is a way 'is another clause'.

Theory of Transformational Grammar: This is one of the most influential of theories of grammar or syntax. There are certain phrase-structure rules. By combining the elements according to phrase-structure rules a sentence with meaning is generated. It includes surface structure and deep pharse structure.

Surface Structure: The basic idea or proposition is expressed in a simple declarative sentence in the surface structure. What is called surface structure is the actual expression of speech in deep-structure organization.

Deep Phrase Structure: When a person intends to communicate a thought, words are grammatically organized is what is known as the deep phrase structure according to the phrase structure rules. Transformation rules change the deep structure into surface structure, thus allowing the same deep structure organization to be expressed in any number of different surface-structure phrases and sentences.

Development of Thinking: The Swiss psychologist, Jean Piaget devised a theory to explain how organization of knowledge occurs. His approach is known as genetic epistemology. Epistemology studies the nature and acquisition of knowledge. The development of knowledge involves assimilation and accommodation apart from genetic origins.

According to Jean Piaget, our thinking processes change radically, though slowly from birth to maturity because we constantly strive to make sense of the world. He identified four factors biological maturation, activity social experiences and equilibration—that interact to influence changes in thinking.

Maturation: It is the unfolding of the biological changes that are genetically programmed, Here, parents and teachers plays a little role.

Activity: Activity is another influence for acquiring knowledge. Physical maturation contributes for activity. When a child's co-ordination is reasonably developed.

For example: the child may discover principles about balance by experiencing with a sea-saw. Thus, we act on the environment as we explore, test, observe and eventually organize information we likely to change our thinking process at the same time.

Social Transmission: As we grow, we interact around us. According to Jean Piaget, our cognitive development is influenced by social transmission or learning from others. Without social transmission it is very difficult to acquire knowledge. The amount of knowledge acquiring by social transmission varies according to stage of cognitive development.

Jean Piaget hypothesized four stages of cognitive development are called sensorimotor, preoperational, concrete operational and formal operational. Piaget believed that all people pass through the same four stages in exactly the same order. These stages are generally associated with specific ages, but these are only general guidelines, not labels for all children of a certain age. Often people can use one level of thinking to solve one kind of problem and a different level to solve another.

Piaget noted that a person may show characteristics of one stage in one situation, but characteristic of a higher or lower stage in other situations.

1. *INFANCY: The Sensorimotor Stage:* This is the earliest period in life. It starts from the birth to till two years. Here, the child's thinking involves seeing, hearing, moving, touching, tasting, etc. During this period, the infant develops object permanence, the understanding that objects exist in the environment whether the baby perceives them or not.

   For example: if we show a toy to infant of less than eight months and then hide it, the child stops looking for it. But a year old child searches for a hidden toy. The search suggests that child has attained object permanence. Apart from this, child also accomplishes goal directed actions. The child also shows the tricks of problem solving.
2. *PREOPERATIONAL Stage (2–7 years):* In preoperational stage, the child has not yet mastered these mental operations but is moving towards mastery. The ability to form and use symbols-preoperational period and moves children closer to mastering the mental operations of the next stage. This ability to work with symbols is known as semiotic function.

   The child's earliest use of symbols is in pretending or miming fashion. Children who are not yet able to talk will often use action symbols.

   For example: pretending to drink from an empty cup. This behavior also shows that their schemes are becoming more general and less tied to specific functions. In this stage, a rapid development in language and symbol system occurs. Between the ages of 2 and 4, most children imbibe the vocabulary of about 200 to 2000 words.

   As the child moves through the preoperational stage, the developing ability to think about objects in symbolic form remains limited to thinking in one direction only or using one-way logic. It is very difficult for the child to "think backwards" or imagine how to reverse the steps in a task. Reversible thinking has a limited role during this period.

According to Jean Piaget, the preoperational children are egocentric is nature. They tend to see the world and the experiences of others from their own viewpoint. Egocentric means children often assume that everyone else shares their feelings, reactions and perspectives.

For example: if a little boy at this stage is afraid of dogs, he may assume that all children share this fear. Egocentrism is also seen in child's language.

For example: young children happily talk about what they are doing even though no one is listening. This is called collective monologue.

3. *CONCRETE Operational Stage (7–12 years.):* Piaget coined the term concrete operations to describe this stage of "hands-on" thinking. The basic characteristics of this stage are the recognition of the logical stability of the physical world, the realization that elements can be changed or transformed and still conserve many of their original characteristics and the understanding of these changes can be reversed.

   This is the stage where systematic reasoning and logical thinking starts.
4. *FORMAL Operational Stage (12 years onwards):* In this stage, the adolescent demonstrates formal operations by hypothetico deductive reasoning. Reasoning and logic are well developed. Child thinks about thinking and uses theories to guide it.

   Another characteristic of this stage is adolescent egocentrism. It means the adolescents just become very focused on their own ideas. They analyze their own beliefs and attitudes.

Relationship with Language and Communication: Language starts with sounds, meanings, words and sequences of words, volume, voice tone, inflection, turn taking rules and at last the sentences. Apart from culture, biological and experiential factors play a vital role in language development. In language, we utilize the stored information to use language as a thought. It uses symbols and grammar to join words into phrases and sentences.

Linguistic Relativity Hypothesis: According to linguistic relativity hypothesis, language can actually determine the thoughts we are capable of having. When we use language as a tool of thought or communication we rely on our linguistic competence. Psycholinguistics is concerned with the behavior of using language and also in the way in which behavior is influenced by language.

Thinking and Language: Levels of thinking depends on how we do conversation. Simple definition may have one kind of thinking and complex meanings which can be understood in more than one way are of the other kind. The study of word and concept meaning is known as semantics.

Denotation Meaning: The generally accepted meaning or a word or concept is mentally represented by collections of features distinguishing that word or concept from all others.

For example: the word 'date', 'president', etc. have straight meanings.

Connotative Meaning: It is the emotional and evaluative meaning of a word or concept. Differences in the connotative meanings of words or concepts are an important source of misunderstanding and failure of communication. Whether a word spoken is sarcastic or humorous depends upon the intention of the speaker.

Syntax: It is the basics of word order. It includes clauses qualifiers and conjunctions.

Pragmatics: It involves the appropriate use of language to communicate.

Metalingustic Awareness: It means understanding about language and how it works becomes explicit.

Nursing Applications: A normal and correct thinking is a great asset for a nurse. To think correctly, nurse should cultivate good thinking habits. She should analyze the facts and come to good decision maker. She should remember that clients have varied thinking based on their philosophy, beliefs and attitudes. Let her emotion not control her thoughts. She has to guard against her own wishful thinking, her prejudices and biases when dealing with patients not without any rational basis if she is not alert. She has to cultivate the habit of suspended judgment by waiting to draw evidence. Contacts with people, discussions, reading good books and literature, sensitivity to language, its forms and the habit of facing the problem are other devices for correct thinking.

INTELLIGENCE AND APTITUDE

One of the purposes of living on this universe is to lead a understanding and quality life. The behavior of people will depend upon his nature of learning and thinking. Thinking includes intelligence. It is a complex and difficult to measure but we can perceive it by observation of behavior.

Definitions

Many psychologists defined intelligence in different ways. Here are some of them.

According to Sternberg and Kaufman (1998) define intelligence as the ability to learn from one's experiences, acquire knowledge and use resources effectively in adapting to new situations or solving problems.

Albert Binet defines "intelligence is a capacity to think well, to judge well and so be self critical". It makes a person capable of receiving and maintaining a mental set. It enables man to reach his destination and judge his own faults.

Wells: Intelligence is the property of recognizing our behavior pattern so as to act better in new situations.

William Stern: Intelligence is the ability to adjust oneself to a new situation.

Wechsler: He said that "Intelligence is the aggregate of global capacity of the individual to act purposefully to think personally and to deal effectively with his environment." Here, it has three dimensions. They are (i) Purpose, (ii) Rational thinking, (iii) Effectiveness in the environment. Intelligence is a capacity to aggregate all these.

Stodord: He defines intelligence is the ability to take activities that are characterized by (i) Difficulty, (ii) Complexity, (iii) Abstractness, (iv) Economy (v) Adaptiveness to a goal (vi) Social value, emergence of originals and to maintain such activities under the condition that demand. Concentration of energy and a resistance to emotional forces.

Nature of Intelligence

Intelligence is expressed in-terms of behavior. This is a pragmatic application. We used to say that a person has behaved intelligently (or stupidly) then it is to say that this person has (or lacks) intelligence.

Intelligence is not a "thing" which one can see, hold, touch, etc.

Instead, it is a way of behaving. People differ in degree of intelligence as well as in the kind, i.e. the different mental abilities they have. A particular behavior of some people is consistently at a high level and we call them that they are having good intelligence. Like wise the typical behavior of others is consistently at a much lower level and they are said to be dull, stupid or significantly lacks in intelligence.

One indication of intelligence is how a person learns. Some people learn well, rapidly and very much in certain areas of behavior, while others do quite poorly in these areas but at the same time do well in others.

Learning is not only the indicator of intelligence but it involves the abilities to solve problems of many kinds. It involves the ability to recognize relationships, to recall, to evaluate, to choose wisely or effectively and to apply the past experiences to present behavioral situations. When a person faces a novel situation or problem and must make some adjustment to it, the adjustment is made in keeping with his level of intellectual functioning. Though he has never faced a similar situation before, the intelligent person is able to deal with it more effectively then is the person who is lacking in intelligence. Intelligent persons are fit for using symbols, abstract thinking, perfect calculating, justify performing tasks, working more in less time and achieving the goal or motto, etc.

One more nature of intelligence is regarding its social value and creative power of intelligence. Intelligence has creative power. Individuals with such power think abstractly and constructively. Hence intelligence means centralized and constructive thinking.

Another nature of intelligence is that it provides resistance to emotions. But psychologists prove that to resist emotions is not the functions of intelligence. By personality test human defense mechanism can be measured. Intelligence has nothing to do with this mechanism.

The other nature of intelligence includes individual difference among persons. It has no organic existence. It is not on object. It is a process of activity. Intelligence is an all inclusive term used to explain human thinking, reasoning, and power of understanding, memory, judgment, organized activities and other work. Just accumulation and storing of knowledge may be called wisdom. But practical application of accumulated knowledge in day-to-day life affairs is true intelligence. Hence, intelligence is what intelligent persons do.

Development of Intelligent Behavior

Behavior of infant is entirely different from an adult. He is neither able to support himself nor is he able to solve his daily problems. He has to depend on his parents and caretakers for everything. He lacks the ability to cope with the environment, which is an essential aspect of intelligence. This evidences that intelligence and cognition of man develops with age.

Thurstone's primary abilities test shows that different abilities grow at different rates; the gain is generally rapid in childhood but slows down is teens. Development of intelligence from birth to 12 years of age is marked by the sensorimotor and physical development of the child. During these years he also shows an increase in his vocabulary, logical thinking and qualitative change. First 12-years of his life make him very similar to an adult from a helpless infant.

In a study, mental ability scores of individuals were found to grow steadily till 20-years of age. In other study some individuals were followed from birth to 36-years to observe the development of intelligence. It was found that the mental ability of few of them continued to increase till the age of 26-years after which it leveled off. After the age of 40 a steady decline in the intellectual ability was observed. It was followed by a sharp drop in intelligence after the age 60. Mental abilities requiring speed and extensive use of short term memory reach their peak between the age of 30 and 40 and decline afterwards. But general knowledge shows little decline with age. Decline in specific mental abilities is related to one's occupation also. It supports the theory or 'use or loose'. According to this theory, more use of certain faculties leads to their better growth during the developmental years while in late adult years and old age it slows down their decline. But this decline in intelligence does not signify descrease in competence of individual as the descrease in speed and efficiency is compensated by his knowledge and experience.

Features of Intelligence

Various definitions and meaning bring forth the following features:

1. Intelligence is an innate mental ability which grows and is influenced by the environment.
2. It shows the capacity to adapt to new or changed situations quickly and correctly.

3. It consists in the ability to carry on the higher mental processes such as reasoning, problem-solving, criticism, application, and judgment.
4. It implies the capacity to learn difficult tasks and the ability to solve increasing difficult problems
5. It shows the capacity to observe relationships and detect absurdities.

CLASSIFICATION OF INTELLIGENCE

Individual Differences in Intelligence

Every individual is unique by nature, intelligence differs among people. Some people learn quickly, some learn very slow. But those who are showing low intelligence, they face a great barrier to fulfill their desires and to attain a high standard of living. Differences in intelligence also greatly affect peoples ability to cope with demands of society. Actually, the intelligence can be scored such as other traits. It is distributed in the population in such a way that most people scores in middle range and very few people mark very high or very low scores. It follows bell shaped distribution or normal curve.

The differences in intelligence may result from one or more of the following factors:

Heredity

The limits of one individual's intellectual development are determined by the genes which he has received from his parents. For example, a chimpanzee cannot achieve the proficiency in language which a human child can.

Physical Health

People with low intelligence have been found to have abnormalities in their brain and in the central nervous system. Thyroid deficiencies or pituitary gland abnormalities retard intellectual development. Birth injuries can result in cerebral anemia and thus cause mental defectiveness.

Environment

It includes child's biopsycho economic status. Favorable environmental conditions encourage the cultivation of that intelligence which they have.

Intelligence Classified/Types of Intelligence

Earlier it is considered that intelligence was a single index of cognitive ability. Now, it is believed that, intelligence is not a single entity rather there are many intelligences. These are displayed by people while solving their day to day problems. Howard Gardner hypothesized the theory of multiple intelligence which is independent of each other. These are:

1. **Linguistic intelligence:** This is related to reading, writing, listening, speaking and understanding language.

2. **Logical-mathematical:** It is associated with the understanding and manipulation of symbols especially those involved in mathematical operations.

3. **Spatial:** Spatial intelligence is used in making mental images and professions like sculptors, engineers, pilots, sailors and divers, etc.

4. **Musical:** This type of intelligence involves sensitivity to pitch and tones of sound.

5. **Bodily-kinesthetic:** This type of intelligence is expressed in the activities like athletics, dancing, surgery and crafts, etc.

6. **Interpersonal intelligence:** It is found in professions that require dealing with other people like sales people, teachers, nurses, religious leaders, etc. They have a good understanding of the motives and emotions of others.

7. **Intrapersonal:** This intelligence is related to understanding of one's own self, feelings and motives.

8. **Naturalistic:** This type of intelligence is possessed by farmers, zoologists, botanists, hunters and tourists, etc. These people show a very good understanding of the flora and fauna and the natural world around them.

Thus intelligence can be called the global capacity to profit from experience and goes beyond the provided information.

Clinical Classification

According to American Psychiatric Association. The intelligence is classified into the following:

Mentally retarded children: People are appropriately regarded as mentally retarded if:

Table 3.1: Classification of intelligence

IQ	Type	% of Population
130 and above	Very superior	2.2
120–129	Superior	6.07
110–119	Bright normal	16.1
85–109	Average	59.1
70–84	Borderline	13.6
55–69	Mild mental retardation	2.1
40–54	Moderate mental retardation	0.1
25–39	Severe mental retardation	0.003
Below 25	Profound	0.0000005

1. They attain IQ's below 70 on an appropriate intelligence scale.
2. Their adaptive skills are inadequate to cope with ordinary daily tasks.

Exceptional Intelligence/Giftedness: An IQ of 130 and above is considered as gifted children or also called as genius. According to Lewis M Terman (1921), a Psychologist at Stanford university has done a longitudinal study on 857 boys, 671 girls had IQ ranging from 130 to 200. The study findings demonstrated that gifted were socially well adjusted and often skilled leaders. They were also above average in height, weight and physical attractiveness. He also has shown that his gifted children were not only not more susceptible to mental illness than the general population. They were actually more resistant to mental illness. Only those with the highest IQs (180 and above) were found to have some social and behavioral adjustment problems as children.

Theories of Intelligence: Intelligence has many factors. To explain the true nature of intelligence, psychologists put forward different theories and thereby they try to demonstrate the organization and function of it. The different theories are:

1. Unitary or monarchic theory
2. Two factor or ecliptic theory
3. Three factor theory
4. Sampling or oligarchic theory
5. Multiple factor theory
6. Group factor theory
7. Hierarchical theory
8. Three dimensional theory

9. Fluid and crystallized theory
10. Intelligence A and Intelligence 'B' theory
11. Sternberg's Triarchic theory

Unitary or Monarchy Theory

Binet, Terman and Stern, are the chief exponents of this theory. According to this theory, intelligence is the sum total of all human capabilities. It is a power or energy which affects all activities of the individual. This is a generalized capacity that enables man to develop in all aspects of life.

This theory is proved weak when a person fails to show expertise of same level in all his works. Measurement of IQ in different types of tasks give different numbers. Hence, intelligence can not be one power or energy that affects all activities of the individual. All activities cannot be affected by intelligence equally. As the theory does not give the comprehensive view, it is rejected.

Two Factor or Ecliptic Theory

Karl Spearman (1904) was the profounder of this theory. By using correlation method, he devised two factors, that is his opinion, intelligence consists of the first factor, symbolized as '§' that is general intelligence, mental ability or common ability and the second 's' that is specific intelligence.

The factor '§' remains the same and unchanged for an individual while's' factor varies from task to task. Individual difference is due to the variation in both '§' and's' factors, while '§' is common for all activities and also essential for every task's' factor varies in degrees and hence performances of an individual in various tasks differ's' factor is inherited and modified by learning, but '§' factor is inherited its ability is fixed. In order to be successful in all activities the '§' factor must be a developed one. But's' factor must be trained and put to habit. To perform a particular task successfully both '§' and's' factors are required and their required quantity depends upon the nature of the task. Hence for different works proportion of '§' and's' different. As the's' factor is accumulated from educational and environmental experiences it is not reflected in all the works equally. The's' factor can be divided in smaller groups. For example, reasoning is included in's' factor, can be divided into abstract or concrete as well as inductive or deductive.

Three Factor Theory of Intelligence:

Spearman added a third factor to his earlier proposed theory and the termed the third factor as 'group factor'. The third factor is less general, widespread and homogenous than 's' factor. Hence human intelligence is the product of the interaction among the three factors:

a. *Sampling or Oligarchic Theory:* Thomson advocated this theory. He divided intellectual abilities into certain groups. These groups are independent of each other. But there is a close relationship between the abilities belonging to the same group. Every group has its own items or subjects. An individual if intelligent in one group, may not be intelligent in another group. But he will show intelligence in the various subjects, that particular group is constituted of.

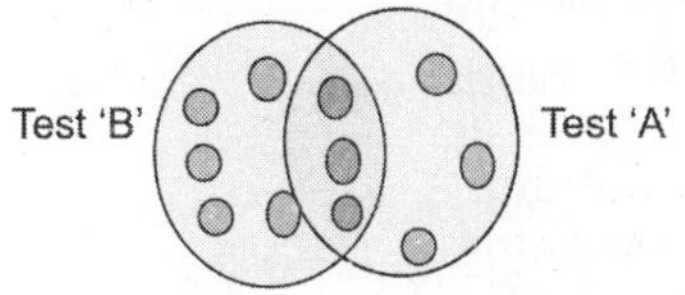

Fig. 3.4: Thomson's theory of sampling

This theory is also called as Thomson's Sampling theory because an individual has to sample out certain important abilities, out of the whole world of his abilities. By sampling he selects one of his mental abilities to perform certain type of work. It is based on correlational technique.

Thomson also accepted 'g' factor or 'general ability' of spearman. But he considered it of second order factor.

Multiple Factor Theory

Multiple factor theory was proposed by EL Thorndike. In his opinion there are some stimulus and mental reactions to them. Every stimulus and its response is different in its nature from another stimulus and its response and its unique nature is called intelligence. According to Thorndike, differences in nerve structure among person is the root cause of individual difference in the field of intelligence. He has developed four criterions of intelligence, i.e. level, span, area and speed.

The Group Factor Theory

This theory is also called as Thurstone's theory of primary mental abilities. According to this theory, intelligence is not the manifestation of some factors or general abilities. Rather it believes in grouping mental abilities. Every group has a prime factor. These primary abilities work independently of each other. These primary abilities put mental and physical abilities into work. There are nine groups of abilities according to this theory. They are:

1. Visual or spatial ability
2. Perceptual
3. Numerical
4. Verbal comprehension
5. Word fluency
6. Memory
7. Inductive reasoning
8. Deductive reasoning
9. *Problem-Solving:* He gave more stress upon general intelligence factor, which could not be subdivided.

Hierarchical Theory

English psychologist Vernon synthesized this theory. He compares the mind to a 'genealogical tree' where 'g' factor is the most prominent component in the sense that it accounts the greatest proportion of differences inabilities. He divided the general mental ability into two group factors known as verbal education factor (v:ed) and practical-mechanical-spatial-physical (K:m) factor while analyzing statistically a third factor named mathematical factor (m) also emerged. The first two or all the three factors can be further divided and subdivided into a number of specific abilities, e.g. vocabulary, fluency, perceptual, speed, scientific and technical abilities, physical ability, etc.

The theory can be represented as follows:

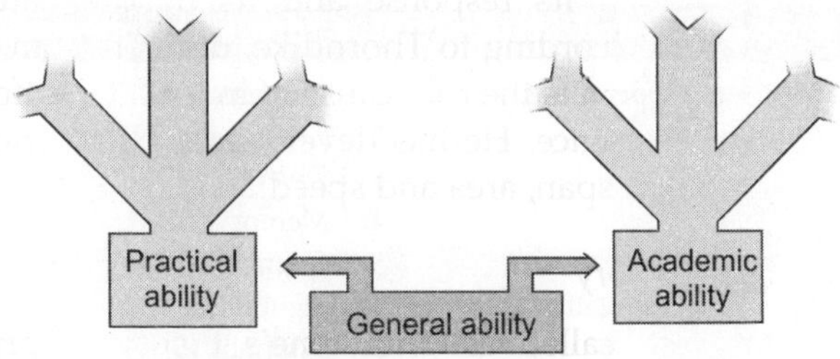

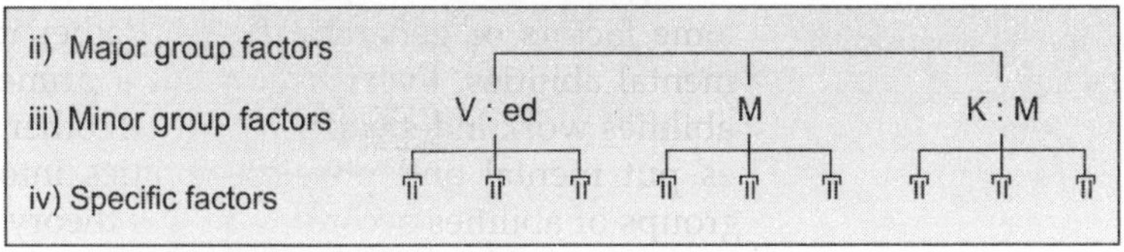

Fig. 3.5: Another way of diagrammatic presentation of the theory (General Mental Ability)

THREE DIMENSIONAL/OR SI MODEL

Guildford and his associates studied on factor analysis and formulated three dimensional models also known as the structure of intellect model (SI). According to him, human intellect can be classified into 120 factors. He opined that there are three basic parameters along which any intellectual activity takes place. These three are operation, product, content. Again there are 5 operations 6 products and 4 contents, from this the total number of factor we get are 6 × 5 × 4 = 120. But Guilford failed to discover all these factors.

For example: A factor MBT means—memory behavioral transformation. A diagrammatic presentation of the SI model is as follows:

a. Fluid and crystallized Theory: Fluid and crystallized theory was sponsored by Cattel. He classifies human intelligence into two categories. The first is fluid intelligence and the second is crystallized intelligence. He also used general ability factor and put emphasis upon general or inherited potentialities and environmental factor. The earlier one is fluid and the later crystallized.

Table 3.2: The systematic detail of this theory gives us the following data

a. Operations	1. Evaluation (E)
	2. Convergent (N)
	3. Divergent (D)
	4. Memory (M)
	5. Cognitory (C)
b. Contents	1. Figural (F)
	2. Symbolic (S)
	3. Semantic (M)
	4. Behavioral (B)
c. Products	1. Units (U)
	2. Classes (C)
	3. Relations (R)
	4. System (S)
	5. Transformation (T)
	6. Implication (I)

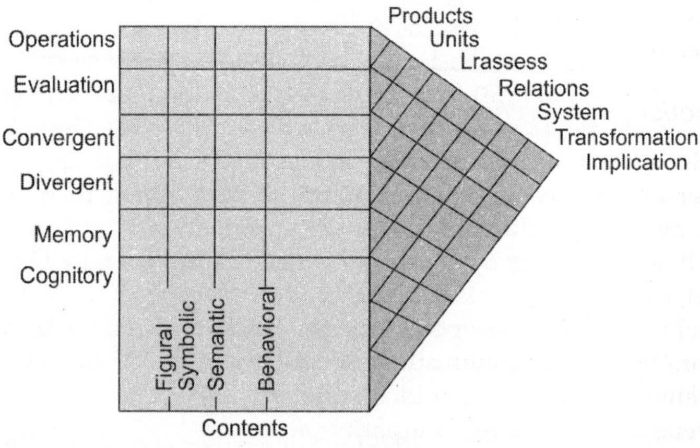

Fig. 3.6: SI Model

Intelligence A and B Theory

Hebb advocated this theory. He says that intelligence 'A' represents the capacity of the central nervous system for forming, retaining and recombining schemata and it is ultimately determined by the genes. Intelligence 'B' represents the cognitive abilities which have been built-up during infancy and childhood, and which do not develop in the absence of suitable environmental stimulations.

Sternberg's Triarchic Theory

Sternberg in 1988 has theorized that there are three kinds of intelligence called the triarchic theory of intelligence. This theory is similar to Aristotle's theory of intelligence is composed of theoretical, productive, and practical aspects.

In Strenberg's theory, the three aspects are analytical, creative and practical intelligence. Analytical intelligence refers to the ability to break problems down into component parts or analysis for problem solving. This can be measured by intelligence tests and academic achievement tests. Creative intelligence is the ability to deal with new ways of solving problems. Practical intelligence is the ability to use information to get along in life. It predicts success in life but has a low relationship to academic or analytical intelligence.

Emotional Intelligence

This was first introduced by Salovey and Mayer (1990) and later expanded by Goleman (1995). Emotional intelligence is the awareness of and ability to manage one's own emotions as well as the ability to be self-motivated, to feel what others feel and to be socially skilled. According to Goleman, emotional intelligence is a more powerful influence on success in life than more traditional views of intelligence. One who is emotionally intelligent possesses avoid of emotions such as anger, impulsiveness and anxiety. Empathy, sensitivity, persistence and the ability to motivate our self also includes an emotional intelligence.

Measuring Intelligence

Intelligence of a person is measured by a standardized scales. These are of the following:

1. Stanford Binet scales: Terman (1916) a researcher at Stanford University, adopted German psychologist William Stern's method for comparing mental age and chorological age (number of years since birth) for use with the translated and revised Binet test. Stern's (1912) formula was to divide the mental age (MA) by the chronological age (CA) and multiply the result by 100 to get rid of any decimal points. The resulting score is called as intelligence quotient or IQ.

$$IQ = \frac{MA}{CA} \times 100$$

For example, if a child who is ten years old (CA) takes the test and scores a mental age of 15 (MA), the IQ will be

$$IQ = \frac{15}{10} \times 100 = 150$$

This test can used to compare the intelligence of different age groups. Used for selection of employees into special education programs.

Flow chart 3.3: Hierarchy of intelligence

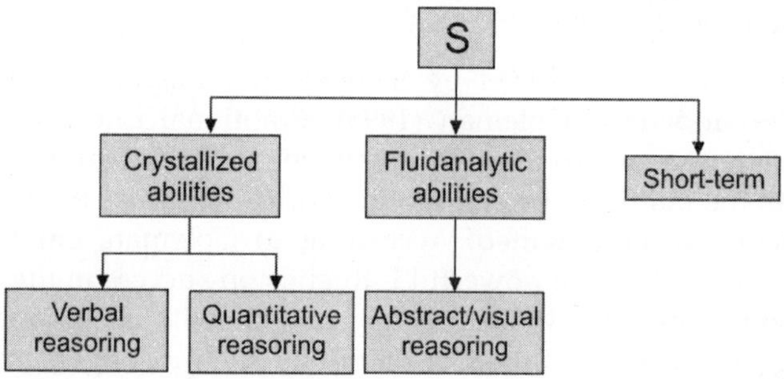

This test is based upon a three level hierarchical model of intelligence. At the top of the hierarchy is 'S' or general intelligence. At the next level is crystallized abilities, fluid abilities (abstract/ visual reasoning) and short-term memory. The third level in the hierarchy falls under crystallized abilities, which are divided into verbal and quantitative reasoning.

2. Wechsler scales: David Wechsler (1991) devised a series of tests for specific age groups. He developed an IQ test specifically for adults. He later designed for school age children, preschool children and also for early graders. The Wechsler adult intelligence scale (WAIS-IV). Wechsler intelligence scale for children (WISC-IV) and the Wechsler preschool and primary scale of intelligence (WPPSI-III) are used now-a-days. These tests have a verbal and performance (nonverbal) scale, tests vocabulary, comprehension and general knowledge, whereas, the performance component scale tests such skills as arranging blocks to match a pattern, identifying a missing parts in pictures, and putting pictures representing a story in order.

Kaufman Scales

The Kaufman assessment battery for children is an individually administered test of intellectual functioning designed for use with children between the ages of 2½ and 12½ years. There are four scales in the Kaufman assessment battery for children. Sequential processing scale, simultaneous processing scale, mental processing composite and achievement scale. The sequential processing scale has three subscales the simultaneous has seven; and the achievement has six. The number of subtests administered depends upon the child's age, ranging from seven at age, two year, six months to 13 at ages, seven and older. A global score is obtained for each of the four scales. The mean of each is 100 and the standard deviation is 15.

Use of Intelligence Tests

These include:

a. For selecting students for admission to various different courses.
b. For classification of student according to their mental ability.
c. For detecting the mentally superior and mentally backward and feeble minded children.
d. For finding out the suitability of students for jobs and career.

e. For vocational selection.
f. For remedial teaching.
g. For rewarding the concessions and scholarship, etc.
h. For clinical evaluation.
i. For research and education.
j. For helping problem children to adjust.

SUMMARY

- Attention is a psychomotor activity which involves the person to concentrate on a specific object or environment.
- Perception involves the integration of sensory information of objects and how we use them in the world.
- Perceptual errors occur because of defect in sense organs. These may be temporary or permanent in nature.
- Learning is a lifelong process. It is perceived as relative permanent change of an individual's behavior or knowledge.
- Learning is formal as well as informal in nature.
- Memory is the process of remembering the past. It involves retentation and sense of recall.
- Recitation and over learning helps to retain memory intact. Forgetting is the part and parcel of memory where the individual fails to recall.
- Thinking is the use of cognitive processes such as perception, mental combinations and resonining.
- Intelligence is the ability to learn and use it in a productive way. Intelligence helps for learning. Favorable health and environmental conditions helps for development of better intelligence . It can be measured by different tests.

TEST YOURSELF

1. Define Attention and clinically differentiate between attention and perception.
2. Enlist the characteristics of learning.
3. What is memory?
4. List out the factors influencing memory.
5. Differentiate between thinking and reasoning.
6. Discuss the nature and use of intelligence.

Chapter 4

Aptitude

APTITUDE

Intelligence is made-up of many abilities. Aptitude usually refers to the ability to learn a particular kind of skill required in a specific situation. It is a particular skill or a potential. While intelligence is a measure of general ability, aptitude is a special ability. It is the special aptness or fitness for a special ability, such as musical, mechanical, artistic, scholastic or religious. It is, highly specific tendency or aptness due to special neural or muscular organization possessed by the individual which sets him apart as being superior to the average in performance in that trait or activity. Different people show different aptitudes for different activities.

Aptitude is neither completely inborn or acquired. It is the outcome of both heredity and environment. Aptitudes are talent potentials but can be improved by training in environment.

Concept of Aptitude

The word 'apt' refers to appropriate justified correct or right depending upon the context. Aptitude usually means potential for achievement. It imbibes that person's performance will increase markedly with extra training if he has an aptitude for a certain matter. Aptitude tests are used to measure the specialized abilities required in specific occupations and activities.

Uses

1. Aptitude tests are used for schooling and professional studies where specific abilities have to be tested which are important to the profession.
2. Vocational aptitude tests are used by employers to select employees.
3. Vocational counselors use vocational aptitude tests to help people assess their aptitudes for different types of work and career counseling.

Type of Aptitude Tests

1. *Scholastic Aptitude Test:* Scholastic aptitude test is used to predict academic success. These tests are used in arts, law, medicine, nursing and allied health sciences.

   For example: The graduate record examination (GRE) test is designed for students of graduates in arts and sciences. The other one is Miller analogies test (MAT) is used to predict success in graduate level.
2. *Vocational Aptitude Tests:* It refers to an assessment about how likely it is that an individual will be successful and satisfied in a particular job given, what is known about his or her interests, abilities training and education, etc.
   a. *Vocational Aptitude Tests for Specific Jobs:* The abilities tested by intelligence and scholastic tests are referred as cognitive abilities. Such abilities are necessary for getting along in school and a certain level of schooling is a requirement for entering certain occupations.
      For example: vocational aptitude tests for mechanics and machine operators measure mechanical ability or the ability to manipulate objects. Different jobs require different combinations of mechanical abilities, so there may be different tests.
   b. *Psychomotor Tests:* Psychomotor tests are also a type of vocational aptitude tests. These tests involve psychomotor tasks such as macular strength, steadiness, manual dexterity, speed of response to a signal and coordination of many movements in a unified whole. For example, differential aptitude test (DAT) is used for counseling

high school and non college students. The scores, either singly or in various combinations can be used to predict scholastic success as well as success in tasks requiring specific aptitudes.

3. *Vocational Interests:* A vocational interest is predicted by following tests:
   a. The strong-Campbell vocational interest Inventory
   b. The Kudler occupational Interest Survey:

Individual Differences and Variability

There are three basic assumptions concerning aptitudes which are justified by observation and studies:

1. An individual's potentialities are not equally strong. There are individual differences among the traits within an individual. Intra individual differences are also seen.
   For example: a person may have good nursing aptitude but very poor writing aptitude.
2. Individuals differ from one another in their aptitude. All people do not inherit the same endowments nor do they developing it easily.
3. Differences among individuals and within individuals are fairly stable. An individual who is definitely superior in a certain kind of aptitude at the age of eight, will as a rules be above average in that kind of aptitude at the age of 18 or 28. Patterns of aptitude do change but a complete reversal is a matter of research.

Aptitude and the Nurse

Nursing requires a certain number of special aptitudes. Manual dexterity is useful in clinicals, speed is useful in all nursing tasks. Linguistic ability makes communication well and easier in examination. Musical aptitude is useful in a nurses own life. Some special aptitudes in sports, music or art may be of great value to nurses in rehabilitating the clients.

A knowledge of the aptitudes, their measurements and conditions will be helpful to the nurse to develop a proper aptitude for her profession and to guide those around her. This will also give her an optimism and contributes for her success in life and profession.

Alternations is cognitive processes

Cognition of the person can be altered by many factors. These are:

a. Drug abuse and Medicines—Drugs like marijuana, LSD, alcohol cause intoxication. The user perceives a variety of alterations in cognitive areas pertain to memory and thinking functions. Acute drug administration alters brain activity.
b. Accident, trauma, shock, etc. can alter the cognitive areas specially attention and memory processes.
c. Ageing—Much of knowledge and skills are gained at later ages of life span whereas losses in memory and reduced ability to think is also noted at later life period.
d. Changes in hormonal level also bring about change in the brain electric activity and this alters the thinking and higher mental functions of the brain.
e. Emotionality in excess also affects the cognitive processes in a negative way so as to give way to alterations.
f. Dyslexia causes alteration in attention and visual functions. This also contributes for alteration is cognitive processes.
g. Pathological condition of the brain is change in anatomic structure shows alteration in the function of the cognitive processes.
h. People with personality disorders like depersonalization and derealization disorder, often report difficulties in perception, concentration and problem solving techniques.

SUMMARY

- In order to perceive an event it must be focused upon. This focus is called attention.
- Perception refers to those processes that give coherence and unity to sensory input.
- Learning is any relatively permanent change in behavior that occurs as a result of practices and experience. Learning is a continuous process from womb to tomb.
- Learning includes thinking and memorization. Memory includes encoding, storage retrieval of what has been learnt.

- Forgetting refers to the apparent loss of information already encoded and stored in long-term memory.
- Thinking consists of the cognitive rearrangement or manipulation of both information from the environment and the symbols stored in long-term memory. Thinking is the set of cognitive processes that mediate or go between stimuli and responses. Thinking and language go through regular stages of development as a child grows. Thinking includes all of the mental activities associated with concept formation, problem solving intellectual functioning creativity, complex learning memory symbolic processing, imagery, etc.
- Intelligence is the aggregate or global capacity of the individual to think rationally, to act purposefully and to deal effectively into the environment.
- Aptitude means potential for achievement. It is an individual who displays his skills and abilities.
- Cognitive processes are assessed by IQ tests and aptitudes tests. In-depth knowledge regarding these tests, helps the nurse to carry out the nursing care very effectively.

TEST YOUSELF

1. Define Aptitude.
2. Differentiate between aptitude and intelligence with an illustration.

Chapter 5

Motivation and Emotional Processes

INTRODUCTION

In a life term human beings survive on motives. Every person wants to achieve a great milestone in a life time. To achieve success they work hard to fulfill their goals. The driving and pulling forces toward success is named as motivation.

Definitions and Meaning

Many theorists are defined the term motivation as follows:

- Petri (1996)—Motivation is the process by which activities are started, directed and continued so that physical or psychological needs or wants are met.
- Baron (2008) defines motivation is an internal processes that cannot be directly observed in the situation but which are real, nevertheless, and which serve to activate, guide and maintain people's actions.
- According to Mc Donald, motivation is a change of a power structure in a human being which is related to stimulus and reaching a goal.
- HW Bernard "motivation refers to all those phenomena which are involved in the stimulation of action towards the particular objective where previously there was little or no movement towards these goals.
- According to Maslow—Motivation is an almost universal characteristic of particularly every orgasmic state of affairs.

Meaning of Motivation

The word motivation is infact from the Latin word "mover" meaning to put into action or to move. So it is the process of arousing movement in the organism. The process that put the individual into physiological or psychological action, and by which man becomes able to fulfill his needs and desires is called motivation. According to Wordsworth, 'motivation is the activity in progress'.

Motivation is a process by which an individual is "inspired", goadded to do something. It is one of the most important conditioning which aid learning and life. This psychophysiological construct impels the individual to achieve his predetermined goal (s). According to Bhatia, he confirms to motivate is to induce movement. Motivation is a broad- based term and encompasses many aspects of behavior. It might be designed as "the tendency for the direction and selectivity of behavior to be controlled by the conditions to consequences and the tendency of this behavior to persist until a goal is achieved". Motivation is purposive, without the presence of goals this process may not start at all. The goal may be biological in nature or purely sociological. A goal is the initiator of the activity in the organisms and once the action is started, it must find some direction and some end. The inspiration to act or react in a particular manner may come from "within" or "outside". A "felt need" is a precondition for motivation. "Need" or "goal" are thickly related. In the absence of other cannot exist.

In work, study or sports, individuals need to be motivated. Without proper motivation no individual would ever strive to respond to the incoming stimuli and adapt to situations. Physiological maturity and psychological readiness are the two essential conditions for learning. An internal condition arousing, sustaining and directing the intensity of efforts is a motive condition. Motives that impel an individual to act in certain way, imply basically two-things, i.e. the drive which is the internal tensioned-state of the organism and the goal which is the final stage of strife. The "will to learn"—"will to strive', and "will to fight", are essential processes of motivation. Motivation is in fact the reinforcer of action. A person who is better motivated is bound to achieve greater success than the one who has not been properly motivated if all other factors are favoring, the former would look more enthusiastic, more lively and over brimming with spirit than the latter.

CONCEPTS OF MOTIVATION

Important concepts about motives includes the following:

1. *Inferences:* Motives are inferences from behavior. Inferences refer to the things that are said and done.
2. *Explanations:* If our inferences about motives are accurate, we have a dependable tool for explanation and evaluation of behavior. We can say that most of our everyday explanations of behavior are given in terms of motivation.
3. *Predictions:* Motives also help us make predictions about behavior. While motives do not tell us exactly what will happen but they provide us an idea about the range of things a person will do.
4. *Types of Motivation:* Motivation begins with drives and ends with adjustments. Motives are the primary factors which influences the motivation.

These are:

1. *Primary Physiological Motives:* These are hunger, thirst, pain, sex, impulse, etc.
2. *Secondary Psychological Motives:* This includes wishes for social status, approbation authority over others, etc.
3. *Social Motives:* These include achievement, power to some extent, aggression, etc. These are learned motives that involve other people.
4. *Motives to know:* Stimulus and exploration needs. This is precisely the reason why children try to explore and find out a lot of things in their surroundings.
5. *Motivates to be effective:* Effective motivation and self-actualization includes motivation. There are motives to be effective. A person who strives to satisfy higher needs for justice, beauty order and goodness is said to be a self-actualized person.
6. *Needs:* A need is a binding that exists between the motive and the drive.
7. *Drive:* Alderman defined "Drive as a psychological mechanism directed towards consummatory reactions, that is, reactions which bring immediate and direct value or satisfaction to the individual such as eating, drinking or scoring a goal."

Primary Drive: These are biological in nature; they arise when instincts of hunger, thirst, love etc. are in operation. They are innate and make survival of possible.

Secondary Drive: These arise as a result of primary drive.

Theories of Motivation

Theories of motivation provides us the understanding about urges, wants, needs, desires, strivings and goals. The different theories of motivation are:

1. Drive theories
2. Incentive theories
3. Opponent process theory
4. Optimal – level theory
5. Maslow's theory
6. Hulls theory
7. Psychoanalytical theory
8. Cognitive theory of motivation
9. Instinct theory of motivation
10. Arousal theory of motivation
11. Self – determination theory.

Drive Theories

Drive theories are also called as "push theories of motivation". It means behavior is 'pushed' toward goals by driving states within the person or animal. In human being, reaching the appropriate goal which reduces the drive state is pleasurable and satisfying. *For example:* The person who is thirsty (drive state) searches for water (goal directed behavior) and if he or she gets water (goal attainment) to quench his thirst, he or she feels satisfied. So according to this theory—motivation is said to consist of a sequence of events that is called as motivational cycle. It includes the following factors:

1. A driving state
2. Goal directed behavior initiated by a driving state
3. Attainment of an appropriate goal and
4. Reduction of the driving state and subjective satisfaction and relief when the goal is reached.

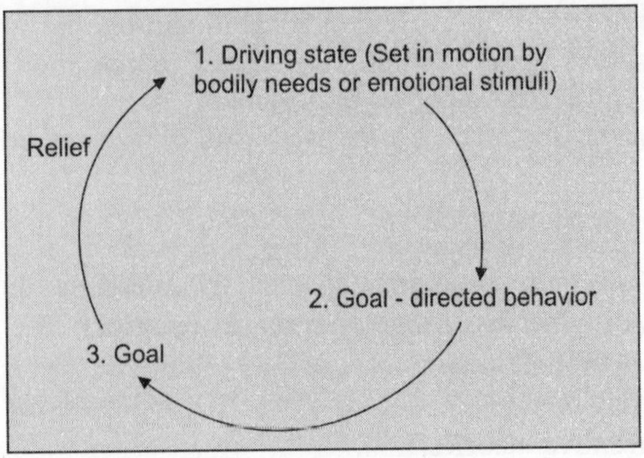

Fig. 5.1: The process of drive (Psychology Munn and Munn)

Incentive Theories

Also called as pull theories of motivation. This is because of certain characteristics the people they already have, the goal objects pull behavior toward them. The goal objects which motivate behavior are known as incentives. The incentive theories idea is that there is something about the goal itself that motivates behavior. The characteristics of the goal can sometimes start a series of motivated behavior. *For example:* A person who wants to win a medal in sports, studies the techniques of winning in a game. The likely reward itself is an incentive.

Opponent - Process Theory

This theory is built on hedonism. Opponent-process theory states that we are motivated to seek goals which give us good emotional feelings and to avoid those resulting in displeasure. It also states that emotional-motivating states are followed by opposing or opposite states. This theory gives a way of thinking about learned motives. Motives are learnt and are not inborn or inherent are known as learned motives.

Optimal-Level Theories

Optimal level theorists, proposes that there is a certain optimal or best level of arousal that is pleasurable. These theories are also called so "just right theories". The individual is motivated to behave in such a way as to maintain the optimal level of arousal.

Humanistic/Maslow's Theory

Abraham Maslow (1954) proposed needs theory. He gave more importance to self-actualization. He postulated that there are several levels of needs that a person must strive to meet before achieving the highest level of personality fulfillment. According to Maslow, self-actualization is the point that is seldom reached at which people have satisfied the lower needs and achieved their full human potential. These were needs both deficiency needs and growth needs. Deficiency needs are needs of the body, such as the need for the food or water, whereas growth needs are for desires like having friends or feeling good about oneself. For a person to achieve self-actualization which is the highest level of growth needs, the primary basic needs must be fulfilled. The figure represents Maslow's series of needs as a pyramid in the

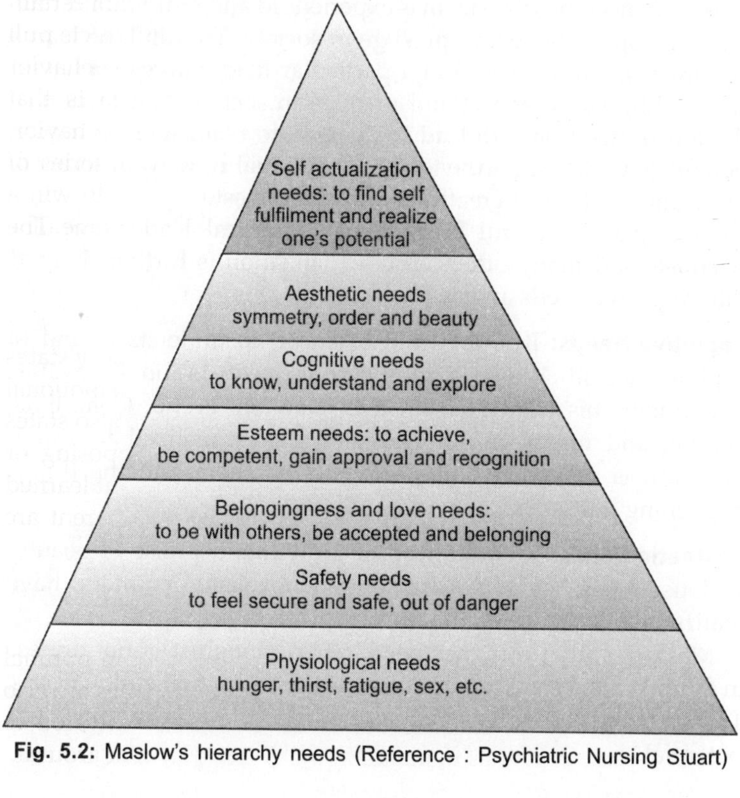

Fig. 5.2: Maslow's hierarchy needs (Reference : Psychiatric Nursing Stuart)

most basic needs for survival at the bottom and the highest at the top. This type of ranking is known as hierarchy.

According to Maslow needs must be fulfilled according to hierarchy. As long as the lower need is not fulfilled upper need in hierarchy cannot be realized. The lowest in order are physiological needs. Every person is born with these physiological needs like hunger and thirst. For survival it is essential to satisfy these needs. Satisfaction of these primary needs leads to realization of second need in order, i.e. safety and security. Individual wants to feel safe and secure in the type of environmental conditions he is living. Surety and guarantee is derived for the satisfaction of physiological needs even for future under safety and security. When the person feels safe and secure their relations with others are needed. Individual wants to relate with others. No one wants to live alone and isolated. Individual wants to live in family and also want better and coordinal relations with others. Thereafter, the fourth need of self esteem is experienced and individual wants to earn respect, fame and prestige in society. To fulfill, he learns specific skills of expertise in a particular field. Success obtained as a result, earns respect and prestige in society. Satisfaction of the fourth need help to lead the person to realization of inborn potentials within the individuals. Individual now want to bring these potentials out in reality to prove him best.

For example: successful businessman, political leader, popular scientists and many others. Self-actualization is further divided into cognitive needs and aesthetic needs.

Cognitive Needs: It is the need to know, to understand and to explore the truth. World famous various scientists and discoveries falls under this need like Einstein, Newton, Freud, Columbus, Darwin and many others. The need theory realized to search the truth is related to the world around them and the things happening in it.

Aesthetic Needs: It is the need of growth and praise of beauty, various poets, singers, dramatists, novelists, painters have realized this need.

Maslow added a higher need, (even though it is not appear in figure) called transcendence above the self-actualization needs. Transcendence involves helping others to achieve their full potential.

Limitations

- Maslow's theory signifies only five types of needs and ignores other various needs, e.g. need of power, need of aggression, etc.

To achieve the highest need, one should satisfy the lower needs. However, in real life it can be cited where lower order needs are skipped and can be achieved the higher level needs.

Hull's Drive Theory

A Hull was a mathematician who formulated the relationship between motivation and performance. He named this theory as mathematico-deducation theory. There are four factors which determine the performance or action of a person. These are drive, habit, probability and inhibition. This can be shown as following:

$$D \times H \times P - I = \text{Performance}$$

Here, **D** means Drive
H means Habit
P means Probability
I mean Inhibition

Drive refers to internal force which pushes the individual toward a particular goal. Habit refers to consistency of some reactions which were successful in achievement of goals in past. Probability is the possibility of achievement in the existing condition.

For example: A student started his studies with full energy and enthusiasm but with the passage of time fatigue and boredom kept on increasing and ultimately he stopped the activity. These all factors vary in degrees and this variability can be calculated in numerical scores. In equation D, H, P is shown as multiplication with each other. Thus strength of performance depends on the scores of D, H and P. As these factors will be raised the strength of performance will also increase. But if any factor amongst D, H and P will be zero, then there will be no performance.

Inhibitory factor I can inhibit the performance. Even if the strength performance is high but the continuous activity will raise the inhibition up to a level where the ongoing activity has to be stopped. As in equation inhibitory factor is subtracted from the product of D, H and P. However, with rest this inhibition will decrease and again the activity can be continued. Hull also explained that need arouses the organism and drive pushes to do activity which help to achieve a goal. Any activity which becomes successful that is repeated again and again. That activity becomes the habit of person.

Hulls theory looks very impressive but lacks the involvement of higher mental functions and also view man to a machine, is not at all justifiable phenomena.

Psychoanalytical theory of motivation

According to Freud, the basic motivating forces that act as drive are embedded in Id and are unconscious. These forces are impulses which are not rational in nature and work on pleasure principle. It shows that the objective of impulses is to seek pleasure. But these impulses of id can not bring the individual in action. Satisfaction of these impulses is based on the sanctions of ego which can channelize energy in human body to any activity. Ego can repress or suppress any impulse from id if it can be harmful or dangerous for the person in reality. Thus ego works on reality principle

Ego not only can bring any impulse in action but can also suppress or repress according to the conditions of the real world. The objective of ego is to satisfy the impulses of id within safe conditions of reality. Impulses of id are also evaluated by super-ego on ethical and moral grounds of an individual. Usually a conflict arises between id and super-ego which should be resolved by ego because ego is rational in nature. Freud introduced the word Libido. It refers to free floating energy within the body of a person. Satisfaction of needs require energy from libido to get the person in action but channelizing of this energy depends upon ego.

Instincts are also considered very important for motivation. Freud gave two types of instincts:

Eros (Life Instincts): It refers to those which motivate a person to live.

For example: hunger, thirst, avoidance of harm and injuries, etc.

Thaneatos (Death Instincts): It refers to those instincts which motivate a person to destroy self to get salvation from the all pains of life. Sometime in the life every person such moments come when he desires to finish himself or to suicide because the miseries of life becomes unbearable. Sigmund Freud's theory is considered a vital for the explanation of motivation but has certain drawbacks. Various concepts such as Id, Ego. Super-ego and libido are all hypothetical in nature which can neither be proved or disproved. Further theory is formulated while working on psychiatric clients and it is not justifiable to apply it to normal people. Basic objective of motivational factor is to have pleasure seeking but it will not be true always.

Cognitive Theory of Motivation

Cognitive theory was propounded by Tolman on the basis of role of higher intellectual functions in motivation. Behavior which took the organism to goal is guided by memory and reasoning. According to Tolman, during goal directed behavior cognitive maps are formed which are used in reaching to the goal.

Instinct Theory of Motivation

This is an old theory to explain motivation on the basis of instincts. Like animals, humans also be governed by instincts. According to Mc Dougall, instinct approach theorists in humans the instinct to reproduce is responsible for sexual behavior and the instinct for territorial protection may be related to aggressive behavior. He has proposed of total of 18 instincts for human including curiosity, flight (running away), pugnacity (aggressiveness) and acquisition (gathering possession).

Arousal Theory of Motivation

Arousal theory expresses an intention on the need for stimulation. A stimulus motive is one that appears to be unlearned but causes an increase in stimulation.

For example: curiosity, playing and exploration. In arousal theory, people are said to have an optimal level of tension. Task performance depends on it. For many kinds of tasks, a moderate level of arousal seems to be best. This relationship between the task performance and arousal is called the Yerkes-Dodson law. However, this effect is modified by the difficulty level of the task. Easy tasks demand a somewhat "high moderate" level for optimal performance, whereas difficult tasks require a "low-moderate" level. Maintaining an optimal level of arousal, may involve reducing tension or creating it.

For example: students who experience test anxiety (high-level of arousal) may seek out way to reduce that anxiety in order to improve test performance. Students who are not anxious at all may not be motivated to study well, lowering their performance. Many theorists of this, believe that the optimal level of arousal for most people under normal circumstances is somewhere in the middle, neither too high nor too low.

Self Determination Theory (SDT) of Motivation

This theory is proposed by Ryan and Decei in 2000. According to them, there are three inborn and universal needs that help people gain a complete sense of self and whole, healthy relationships with others. The three needs are autonomy or the need to be in control of one's own behavior and goals (i.e. self determination), competence or the need to be able to master the challenging tasks of one's life and relatedness or the need to feel a sense of belonging; intimacy and security in relationships with others.

Ryan, Decei, their colleagues believe that satisfying these needs can best be accomplished if the person has a supportive environment in which to develop goals and relationships with others. Such satisfaction will not only foster healthy psychological growth but also increase the individual's intrinsic motivation, which is the type of motivation in which a person performs an action because the act itself is rewarding or satisfying in some internal manner.

Motives and Behavior

Motives

A motive can be defined as a state of arousal that impels an organism to action. It is a rationalization justification or excuse that a person gives as the reason for behavior. Motives can be either inherent, biological motives or learned, like social motives.

FEATURES OF MOTIVES

1. Motives cannot be observed directly. We infer their existence from what people say about the way they feel and from observing that people work toward certain goals.
2. We may not be aware or conscious of our own motives. Hence, behavior can be driven by unconscious motivation.
3. Motives help us to make prediction about behavior.

MOTIVES AND BEHAVIOR

Biological Motives

The basic of biological motives is mostly in the physiological state of the body. The body tends to maintain a state of equilibrium called homeostasis. Many biological motives are triggered, in part, by departures from balanced physiological conditions of the body. The following are some of the physiological motives that have considerable influence on our everyday life:

1. Hunger
2. Thirst
3. A desire for sex
4. Temperature regulation
5. Sleep
6. Pain avoidance
7. Need for oxygen.

Hunger

The basic motive necessary for life primarily is hunger. This biological motive may be initiated when the blood levels or rates of use of nutrient substances fall below a certain point glucose or blood sugar and free fatty acids are among the important nutrients in the blood which may be involved in hunger motivation. The cessation of hunger motivation is related to nutrient receptors in the stomach which provide 'stop eating' signals and possibly to the release of hormones called cholecystokinin. The parts of hypothalamus—the lateral hypothalamus and the ventromedial have long been considered as brain regions that are important in the regulation of hunger motivation. Some early research indicates that the lateral hypothalamus was a feeding center while the ventromedial hypothalamus is the satiety center. Hypothalamic centers are involved in monitoring the body's fuel supplies the control of metabolism and the perception of food related stimuli.

Thirst

Local stimulus theory predicts that dryness of lips triggers thirst drive but again it cannot be the strong factor to regulate high drinking behavior. It is proposed that conservation mechanism related to maintaining balance of water in the body might be related to arousal of thirst drive. When water deficit takes place in the body, it results into dehydration or special nerve cells called osmorecptors in the hypothalamus. This stimulation triggers thirst drive and drinking behavior. Thirst triggered by loss of water at osmorecptors in hypothalamus is called cellular dehydration thirst. Descrease in volume of water in blood results in hypovolemia. This change in blood releases an enzyme renin that helps in formation of a substance angiotension in blood. This substance can arouse thirst drive. Thus, cellular dehydration at hypothalamus and hypovolemia in blood are two conditions which are responsible for arousal of thirst drive and drinking behavior. It is called double-depletion hypothesis. Further, drinking behavior is stopped when sufficient quantity of intake of water takes place which is signaled by the continuous drinking activity of mouth and dehydration in the body.

Sex

From a physiological stand point, sexual motivation depends to a large on sex hormones. The activation of sexual motivation in humans seems to be controlled more by external stimuli and learning than by hormones.

Social Motives

Social motives are learned from society during life span. These are important for existence in a society. These motives are not cyclic in nature. Achievement of goal does not stop the search for other goal. In need for achievement, individual does not stop efforts to achieve more other goal for success in society. Social motives differ in degrees in different individuals and dominant motives becomes traits of personality.

For example: need of power can add dominance, skillfulness is manipulation of others in personality of a person. The following three motives are predominant in social motives:

- Need for achievement
- Need for affiliation
- Need for power.

Need for Achievement

The need for achievement is a motive to accomplish things to be successful in performing tasks. People high in need for achievement prefer to work on moderately challenging and moderately risky task which promise success on tasks where their performance can be compared with the performance of others. They like to work in situations where they have control over the outcome.

Need for Affiliation

The need for affiliation is a motive to establish, maintain and repair relations. These people look out for opportunity to be with friends as much as possible. They make more phone calls, visits, seek approval and dislike disagreements with strangers. They want to be in the good books of the authority figure.

Need for power

Power motivation is a social motive in which the goals are to influence, control, persuade, lead charm others and enhance one's own reputation in the eyes of other people. These kinds of people may participate in competitive sports, may sometime join association and tries to influence their strength.

Human Aggression

While it has a biological basis, human aggression is primarily under the control of social factors. Hostile aggression in any form of behavior directed toward the goal of harming or injuring another living being who is motivated to avoid such treatment. Among the environmental and social causes of human aggression are:

a. Frustration that is intense, arbitrarily imposed
b. Insults
c. Social pressures and compliance with it
d. Environmental conditions those are unpleasant, such as high temperatures, intense noise and over crowding.

Explorative Motives

These are called as motives to know. Motives to know and to be effective are motives to seek variety in stimulation, to process information about the world around us, to explore and to be effective in measuring challenges from the environment.

Stimulus and Exploration Needs: People spend time, effort and money just to look at things, travel and explore the environment. Stimulus needs and the need to explore are largely behind these activities. What satisfied our stimulus and exploration needs once may not always be constant that way and seek something new. We tend to seek out and prefer stimuli that are both novel and complex. A novel stimulus is one that is somewhat different from what we expect; a complex stimulus is one which contains a great deal of information for us to process.

Effectance Motives

There are motives to be effective. These are called effectance motives.

Effectance motivation: The stimulation and exploration needs can be considered to be involved in attempts to be competent in dealing with the environment. The motivation behind these competence activities has been called as effectance motivation—general motive to act competently, effectively when interacting with the environment.

Intrinsic motivation: It is defined as a person's need for feeling competent and self-determining in dealing with his environment. It is called intrinsic because the goals are internal feelings of effectiveness, competence and self-determination.

Self-actualization: The motive of self-actualization is related to effectance motivation and intrinsic motivation. Self-actualization refers to an individual's need to develop his or her potentialities the fullest use of their capabilities.

UNCONSCIOUS MOTIVES

The motives behind some of our unconscious behavior may be due to unconscious motives that operate in unconscious motivation. It is defined as motivation that is not in the conscious awareness of the person. Not all motivated behavior can be seen as the result of rational, the conscious or the willful. Some of our behavior may be motivated by unconscious factors.

For example: stopping the car when accident triggers and helping with curiosity.

CONFLICTS AND FRUSTRATION

All people wants to live happily and enjoy the life. But, the way to achieve this is not always smooth. Our needs cannot always be adequately satisfied in all situations. We have to face negative and hostile situations. Inspite of these, we have to develop feelings and security, worth and competence. There are restrictions and laws imposed by self and society. It means, there are a variety of barriers or obstacles to satisfy our needs. These barriers and obstacles cause frustration and produce anxiety. Thus frustration is the thwarting of one's desire or need. It refers to failure to satisfy a basic need of conditions, either in the individual or external obstacles. Thus, frustration is a negative feeling when one is prevented from reaching a goal.

Frustration is the interference with the environment of a goal. It is a state of strong emotional tension due to blocking of impulses, if it is continued over prolonged period, it gives rise to psychological disorders.

Source of Frustration

1. *Environmental forces:* These block motive fulfillment. The obstacle may be physical or social, e.g. lack of money, locked door, social obligation.
2. *Personal inadequacies:*
   For example: Disability
3. *Conflicts with other people:* When people lack power and security, conflicts will arise.
4. *Economic deprivation:* Poverty induces conflicts because of unfulfillment of desires.

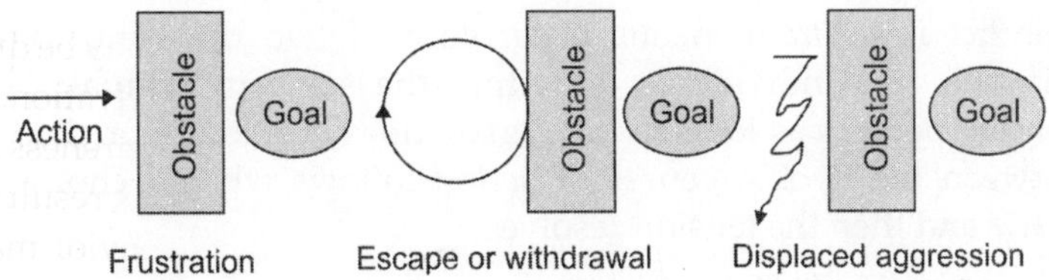

Fig. 5.3: Different processes of frustration (Psychology: Sharma)

5. *Social custom, tradition, religion and taboos:* These laws and codes may, at one time or another interferes seriously with our desires or interests.
   For example: there are laws for hostelites, laws of marriage. These laws and restrictions may be frustrating to some individuals seeking to achieve their personal goals.
6. *Conflict within the individual:* There is a conflict and the solution lies only in thwarting two of our motives and the fulfillment of the third one.

Reactions To Frustration

Frustration creates uncomfortable emotional tension and so the individual tries to reduce the tension in a variety of way. The reactions formed by frustration are as follows:

Direct Approach: Two direct methods of overcoming obstacles are enhancement of effort and changing the mode of attack. If both the methods fail, the third alternative is in changing the goal to one that is more attainable.

Feelings of Inferiority: When increased effort and variation of attack fail and, substitute goals are unavailable, individual often react by developing feelings of helplessness and inadequacy. This emotionally distressing state of the mind is referred to as inferiority complex. It is the form of self-criticism usually involving fear of social disapproval. The common reaction is fear of competition, extreme sensitivity to criticism, suspicion, envy, self-consciousness, worry and extreme self analysis.

Aggressiveness: Aggressive reaction is very common when some external obstacle is the cause of frustration. The target of attack is usually some other person or object and the intensity of attack is proportionate to the amount of frustration.

Types of Conflicts

Conflict is a simultaneous occurrence of two opposing ideas between two individuals or within the same individual. The conflict persists as long as the person does not decide or choose between the two. A course of action follows when a choice is made and then the tension resolves.

Kinds of Conflict

These are:

i. Motivational conflict
ii. Mental conflict
iii Other types of conflict

Motivational Conflict

Motivational conflict results from the simultaneous occurrence of desires which cannot be achieved. It is convenient to analyze this kind of conflicts in term of two kinds of behavior toward goals: approach and avoidance. In connection with positive, desired goals there is an "approach gradient" in connection with negative, repellent goals there is an "avoidance gradient".

Approach – Approach Conflict: It occurs between two positive goals that are equally attractive. The person is attracted at the sametime by two goals that are incompatible.
For example: a person is both hungry and sleepy at the same time.

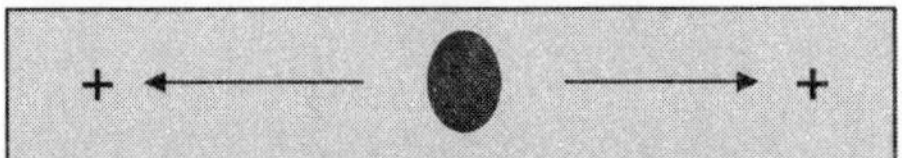

Approach – approach conflict

Avoidance – Avoidance Conflict: It takes placc when one is forced to choose between two negative goals. An individual is caught between two threats, fears or situation that are equally repelling. *For example:* one has to choose between a toothache and going to a dentist. Another avoidance conflict is between unhappy employment and loss of income. These conflicts are not resolved quickly but often go on for a long-time.

The avoidance conflict is the worst type of conflict and is stressful. It leads to indecision, vacillation, inaction and sometimes "freezing", and 'escape' leaving the field.

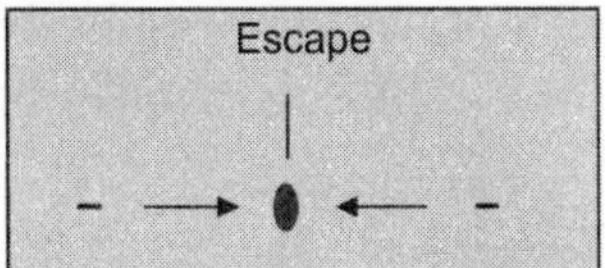

Avoidance - avoidance conflict

People in avoidance—avoidance conflicts, may try different means of running away. They often rely on imagination to free them from the fear and anxiety generated by the conflict. They may spend much time in day dreaming; conjuring up an imaginary world where there are no conflicts or they may recreate in their minds the carefree world of their childhood before the unpleasant tasks and avoidance-avoidance conflict existed. This way of leaving the conflict is called regression.

Approach-Avoidance Conflict: It is most difficult to resolve because in this conflict, a person is both attracted and repelled by the same goal object.

For example: Ice-cream is delicious to eat, but causes obesity.

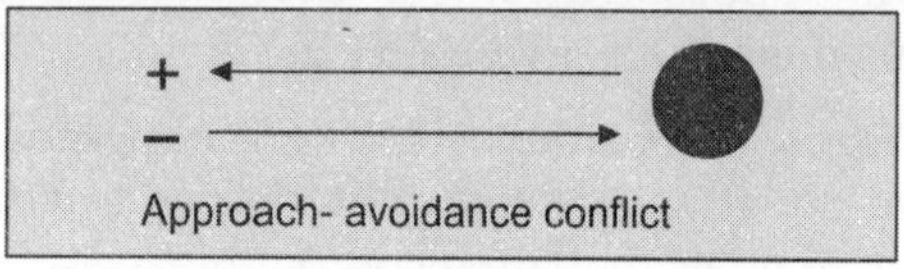

Approach- avoidance conflict

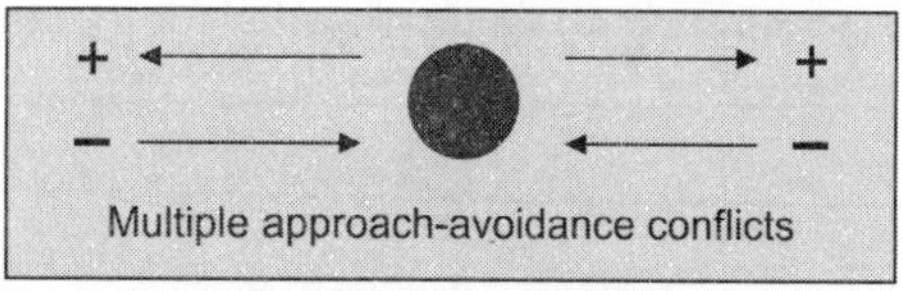

Multiple approach-avoidance conflicts

Multiple-Approach – Avoidance conflicts: Many of life's problems involve many positive and many negative goals.

For example: A man may be in conflict not only about whether to get married but also about which of the several girls would make the ideal wife. Internal obstacles are harder to resolve than the external ones.

People may find ways to getting around environmental obstacles but they find it very hard to escape from obstacles within themselves, i.e. from personal inadequacies and conflicts between motives. The emotional reactions due to approach-avoidance conflicts in which internal obstacles are involved cause several behavioral problems. Conflicts are resolved through the use of certain methods of thinking and acting which either eliminate the conflict or reduce it's severity by using mental mechanisms.

Mental Conflict: Conflict is an essential factor in most frustrating situations. It involves an insurmountable obstacle, the inability to overcome it, a sense of defeat as well as feelings of stress and strain. This implies a conflict between a drive and an obstacle. There may be two or more opposing desires or motives in an individual. Each is clamoring for satisfaction. The individual cannot decide which should be satisfied, a state of tension follows. This inner state of the mind characterized by tension as a result of the simultaneous presence of mutually exclusive or opposing tendencies, impulses or desires is described as mental conflict. The state of tension makes it difficult for the person to choose or to make decision. He hesitates or vacillates between two or three courses of action; sometimes he cannot decide at all. Generally the state of tension or indecision is followed by a course of action. The conflict is present as long as the individual does not decide or as long as he wavers. Thus, it is the state of tension or indecision occurring before a course of action is decided upon.

Other Types of Conflict: These may be a conflict between two persons or between a person and his environment or within the person himself.

Interpersonal Conflict:
For example: Conflict between parents and children.

Intrapersonal Conflict: Conflict between person and his surrounding environment.

Internal Conflict

The conflict within a person, of motives, desires and impulses is called the internal conflict. According to Lewin, these are three types:

i. In which two goals are desired at once, but in which simultaneous attainment of the two is impossible. For example, a student nurse may have a desire to witness a match in the evening and at the same time, may like to go to movie. A student may be caught between two beliefs. He may believe on the hand that the universe is being controlled by mind and spirit and on the other hand, may think that the universe is controlled by mechanical processes. One belief opposes the other.
ii. An individual who wants and does not want a certain object. *For example:* A girl who has passed the examination with science wants to join Nursing college, but at the same time she does not want to join it.

iii. In which an individual does not want to do a thing but is forced to do it.

There are two negative forces causing conflicts.

For example: A student hates to work on an assignment but also dislikes the consequences of not doing it. Student wants to avoid both the things if possible.

Sigmund Freud explained the process of the conflict within a person. It arises at consciousness, the preconscious and the unconsciousness—constitute the process of conflict.

a. When we are aware of the conflict and the sources causing it, the conflict is and to be at conscious level.
b. Preconscious is a unconscious object ready to become conscious. Not imagined or verbalized at a given time, but capable of being imagined. Here, unconscious means mental processes that are only temporarily absent from the mind and can be recalled by effort.
c. When we are not aware of the real motives causing conflict we experience feelings of stress, strain and anxiety. Conflicts at the unconscious level or endopsychic conflict are responsible for such feelings.

The Unconscious Conflict

The mental conflict below the level of conscious awareness is called the unconscious conflict. Most of our emotional disorders are caused by unconscious conflicts. The conflict, even at the conscious level, is a painful affair which creates anxiety in the mind. It should end as soon as possible. It can be ended by following the Id impulses and by ignoring the claims of the ego and superego. Another way of ending the conflict is by throwing these impulses into allied channels sanctioned by society and thus obtaining for them a vicarious satisfaction.

For example: Many women do not marry, and becomes nurses by directing their energies to the care and welfare of children. Unconscious conflicts are often the result of early childhood experiences which have long been forgotten. They follow the process of 'repression' and the formation of 'complexes'.

Repression

It is difficult to endure the idea of defeat which results from the denial of our Id desires. Again, the Id impulses cannot be satisfied in the face of social opposition, nor is it easy to adapt them to other socially sanctioned channels. We need suitable potentialities, education, guidance and environment for that. Normally, the conflict is resolved or ended in an average individual by actually suppressing these wishes into the realm of the unconscious. This unconscious forgetfulness of the Id impulses or throwing down of these impulses into the unconscious is called repression. Thus 'what is unpleasant', obnoxious, embarrassing is banished from consciousness, with repression the conflict shifts from the conscious into the unconscious.

Complexes

The repressed wishes or desires remain active in the unconscious regions of our minds. They slowly gather strength by making alliance with other allied repressed experiences; thus forming an active group. This group of repressed desires work to a common end. This is called a complex. As soon as complexes are formed, they give rise to a conflict in the unconscious, know as the endopsychic conflict. These complexes are just like exiles whose presence back in the conscious is not tolerated. But they do strive to regain consciousness. The forces of the ego and superego would not permit this. If they reverse to the conscious, they would again create conflict and tension.

Censor

The mental force that keeps the repressed undesirable wishes confined to the unconscious region of the mind is technically known as the censor. It is a part of our personality. It represents the moral and social aspects of the ego and superego. During excitement and sleep, the censor weakens. It is during such moments that the repressed wishes seek to regain consciousness. At times, they may come masked or in disguise and thus elude the vigilance of censor. Such disguises may take the form of dream, slips of tongue, active forgetfulness or mannerisms of speech. Sometimes they may manifest themselves in mental mechanisms such as transference, projection, identification, rationalization and others.

Conflict Resolution

Vacillation is very common in all kinds of conflicts. Vacillation means moving forward and backward. If we have insight into own conflicts and the internalized obstacles which create them, we will most likely be more content and less stressful in our lives. Individual has to make positive efforts and alternative option to overcome conflicts. It is very difficult to get a perfect answer for everything in life. So, instead of whatever decision we take, we have to work toward making that decision the most suitable one in accordance with personal aim and societal standards.

Nursing Perceptives

In depth of knowledge about motivation and conflicts, helps to deliver a better care. She has to stay motivated from within. Knowing the purpose of life, nurse can serve better. Whenever client behaves inappropriately, nurse should understand the motive behind it. So that she can try different ways of fulfilling one's motives in a socially approved manner. Nurse can motivate client to recover faster by encouraging them of their progress in the stages of recovery. Even small appreciation will go a long way. Motivation to be rather permanent must be continuous and also consistent. Nurse should motivate herself and others for early recovery.

Emotions and Stress

Can you imagine life without emotions-without joy, anger, sorrows or fear? What would such an existence be like-a life without any feelings? Without emotions life will be dull and standstill. Emotions are the basic feelings of expressions in life. Emotions can activate, motivate and directs the behavior. Emotions are the powerful motive for healthy life.

Emotion Defined

- The Oxford English Dictionary defines emotion as "any agitation or disturbance of mind feeling, passion; any vehement or excited mental state".

- Gates defined emotions are episodes in which the individual is moved or excited.
- According to James Drever defined as emotion is a complex state of organism involving bodily and mental changes and marked by strong feelings.
- PT Young defined as emotion is an acute disturbance of the individual as a whole. Psychological in origin, conscious experience and visceral functioning.
- In the words of Saundra, emotion can be defined as the "feeling" aspect of consciousness, characterized by a certain physical arousal, a certain behavior that reveals the feeling to the outside world and an inner awareness of feelings.

Components of Emotion

Emotions involve two components, i.e. conscious experience and bodily changes. In conscious experience, the person is aware about the kind of emotions he is undergoing.

For example: A person in anger knows that he is angry. Conscious experience takes place in cerebral cortex. Bodily changes involves different type of physiological changes taking place within the body during emotions like change in heart rate, respiratory rate, changes in blood sugar level, etc. These physiological changes depend upon the functioning of sympathetic nervous system.

Perception of emotional situation is also very important in the emotions because same environmental conditions can not arouse emotions similarly in different persons.

For example: An ox running away from person may not arouse him but suddenly if it turns back, the person will be more fearful. Thus, how we perceive the situation plays role in behavior.

Strong emotions can block the reasoning and rationalization of people. Various strange and irrational behaviors can be observed during the excitement.

For example: A patient in extreme fear will react very absurdly with others and can become aggressive toward those who are taking his care.

Changes in Emotions

Internal Changes

During an intense emotional phase most of the bodily changes result from activation of the sympathetic nervous system. These changes are:

1. Increase in blood pressure and heart rate
2. Rapid respiratory rate
3. Dilatation of the pupils
4. Electrical resistance of the skin decreases
5. Blood sugar level increases to provide more energy
6. Clotting of blood in wounds become quicker.
7. Motility of the gastrointestinal tract decreases or stops entirely; blood is diverted from the stomach and intestines and sent to the brain and selected muscles.
8. Hair of the skin are raised causing 'goose pimples'.

External Changes

Cues means hints or clues to know something. Even if we are not speaking in words about our feelings, many a time's external cues are given away by our:

1. Facial features like smile, twisted nose, raised eyebrow, etc.
2. Body posture or poise
3. Tone, pitch of the voice
4. Eye contact
5. Shake hand style
6. Stability of bodily movement.

These are the external cues very well known as 'body language'.

Theories of Emotion

Many theorists described the emotions on the mechanism of its origin and its experience at conscious and bodily level. The following theories describe the emotions in detail.

Cannon Bard Theory of Emotion

Physiologists Walter Cannon (1927) and Philip Bard (1934) theorized that emotional experience and physiological changes occur simultaneously.

For example: On confronting a snake, the running and feeling of fear will take place at the same time.

Cannon gave importance to the role of thalamus, however Bard replaced thalamus with hypothalamus. Sense organs receive the stimulation from emotional situation which is received by hypothalamus. It functions as a relay station and sends the stimulation to cortex and different parts of body at the same time from different nerve pathways. Thus the emotional experience at cortex and physiological changes in different body parts takes place simultaneously.

Cannon and Bard explained that when stimulation reaches to thalamus emotional tone is added to it and later on cortex evaluate its emotional value. Cortex can inhibit some emotional stimulation but if the emotional stimulation is strong it can break the inhibitory control of cortex and emotional experience is observed.

Schachter - Singer Theory of Emotions

This theory is called as cognitive arousal theory. According to this theory, two things will happen before emotion occurs. The physical arousal and labeling of the arousal based on cues from the surrounding environment. These two things happen at the same time, resulting in the labeling of the emotion.

For example: If a person comes across a snarling dog while walking, the physical arousal (increased heart rate, eyes opening wide) is accompanied by the thought (cognitive) that this must be fear. Then and only then will the person experience the fear emotion.

Lazarus and Cognitive Mediational Theory

This theory is proposed by Lazarus in 1991. This theory emphasis more on the aspect of any emotional experience is how the person interprets or appraises, the stimulus that causes the emotional reaction. To mediate means to 'come between' and in this theory the cognitive appraisal mediates by coming between the stimulus and the emotional response to that stimulus.

James Lange Theory

According to this theory, felt emotion is the perception of bodily changes. Our perception of the reaction is the basis for the emotion we experience. So the emotional experience, which is felt emotion, occurs after the bodily changes. This means bodily changes occur first and then the emotional experience follows:

Event ⟶ ? Arousal ⟶ ? Interpretation ⟶ ? Emotion
(accident) (Increased BP, Respiratory rate) (anxiety)

Facial Feedback Theory of Emotion

This theory was originated by Charles Darwin (1898). He stated that facial expressions evolved as a way of communicating intentions, such as threat or fear, and that these expressions are universal within a species rather than specific to a culture. He also believed that when such emotions are expressed freely on the face, the emotion itself intensifies means that the more one similes, the happier one feels. The facial feedback hypothesis assumes that facial expressions provide feedback to the brain concerning the emotion being expressed, which in turn not only intensifies the emotion but also actually causes the emotion.

Activation Theory of Emotions

This theory was proposed by Lindsley (1951). He tried to explain the emotion with the arousal level. Arousal of cortex of a person depend upon the stimulation of reticular formation (RF) is a structure, which makes all organism alert about particular stimuli and produce a general arousal. RF is not only involved in developing arousal, but it also activates the behavior and maintains it till the satisfactions of the goal. RF on brainstem has excitatory and inhibitory connection with the motor neurons of spinal cord, through which it controls the activities of muscles. Projections from RF to cerebrum are very important as these maintain the stimulation for cortical functions. If this reticulocortical arousal mechanism is destroyed, EEG synchronization and behavior somnolence is observed, but it if is stimulated, arousal in behavior is observed. Research shows that if cortical areas are stimulated, changes in the function of RF on brainstem are also observed. It is also found that RF can also develop changes in sensory inputs. Thus Lindsley concluded that RF has a control on muscular activities, critical functioning and also sensory inputs, through which it controls different behaviors of organism.

Motivation and emotions are considered as higher arousal states. Lindsley also considered ascending reticular activating system (ARAS). ARAS is spread over a gray matter, pons, midbrain and diencephalons. ARAS receives sensory inputs from various sensory pathways. This structure stimulates higher brain centers to keep the arousal state of brain. ARAS can also widely stimulate hypothalamus, so that stimulation can reach to any emotion center. Lindsley observed that electrical stimulation of ARAS could develop similar EEG patterns as observed in emotions. Lindsley's findings also showed that neural centers, which control the emotions, are present in brain stem reticular formation (BSRF). It plays an important role in modulating the emotions.

The major function of ARAS is to keep the brain in awakening state. More the ARAS is stimulated higher will be the arousal or activation in organism. If ARAS is calm, then cortical functioning will be lowest kind and the person will feel sleepy. Sensory inputs passes through ARAS, where these are either inhibited or facilitated. Those sensory inputs, which are inhibited at ARAS, never reach cortex and the person never gets aware of that information. Sensory inputs, which are facilitated gets spread over the projection areas on cortex and person starts to aware about that information. ARAS alerts the cortex to receive these outer sensory inputs. This effect is called arousal reaction. Neural impulses from cortex itself can stimulate ARAS. Thus, ARAS can be stimulated by external as well as internal stimulation.

Lindsley described that activation/ arousal of cortex varies at different times. Sometimes it is highly aroused and other times too low. If this arousal is represented on a continuum, then it has two opposite poles. That pole which represents heightened arousal state show strong emotions like aggression. The other pole which represents lowest state of arousal shows sleep or Death. In between these two poles different level of cortical arousal can be represented. On this continuum a point can be marked before which the arousal is non emotional and just after that it gets emotional. After this point as the arousal level rises emotions become more intense and strong-up to the point that behavioral blindness can be observed. The behavior gets totally disorganized. When the arousal level of a person in at zero, then he is in sleep. Cortex is at minimum activation. EEG of that person shows a simple and slow electrical activity. Muscles at this arousal level are in total resting position and send very few impulses to central nervous system.

When a person is in emotional situation, his EEG show high level functioning of cerebra. Cortex is in complete awakening state and reactive to stimulation. When the arousal level is in between the two poles of continuum, the behavior remains highly organized but as soon as, it shifts toward the poles in either direction, falls down in performance is observed. For example, a person who is suddenly wakes-up at night on the ring of phone.

He was ordered by boss to leave immediately for hill station to an urgent task. He decided to go there on his own car, but it was his first drive in hilly areas. So with rise in arousal level, his cortical functioning and muscular activities comes in to higher alertness. In the way, when some sharp turns were experienced, the hypothalamus also gets stimulated, by stimulation from reticular formation. Hypothalamus amplifies the arousal level he started to loose control on the car. This example shows, how the rise in arousal level, effects the behavior of a person. When the person was sleeping, the arousal was at the zero level. Cortical and muscular activities were at the minimum stage. As soon as he wakes-up and come to know about the task from office, the rise in arousal level makes him active. Further, the drive in hilly areas further increases his alertness because of increase in situation RF. However, dangerous turns in the way further enhances the stimulation and the rise in arousal level. Here, RF also stimulates hypothalamus, which amplifies the arousal level and disorganization in cortical and muscular functioning was felt.

Drawbacks

- Lindsley's theory lacks in explanation about strong emotions like aggression which are not based on higher arousal state.
- Lindsley's did not differentiate between emotional and non-emotional behaviors.
- No differentiation between emotion and motivation.
- Perception plays important role in emotions. The same situation can be reacted differently by two individuals.
- This theory has no significance to perception in emotions.

Arnold's Theory of Emotion

Arnold believes that the cognitive processes of an individual interpret his feelings and controls the behavior toward these feelings. Individual first receives the stimulus situation. This perception is categorized as bad, indifferent and good. If the stimulus is good if will be received as bad is rejected and indifferent ignored. Evaluation of a stimulus is not simply based on memory, past experiences but also whether it is bad or good. This evaluation is immediate and it takes place before physiological changes, and emotional experience.

For example: If a person is having a picnic time at some place and suddenly saw a bull coming towards him. He will evaluate the situation using memory and past experience and if find the coming of bull dangerous will experience physiological changes and feeling of fear. Then he will move away from the place. So perception of situation is very important step in emotions. Arnold believes that physiological changes and emotional experience both are determined at cortex.

However, this theory also having certain limitations. Like other theories, it does not explain the role of different parts of brain and the physiological mechanism is not fully determined.

Emotional Adjustment

Emotional adjustment is required because of the constant presence of multiple internal and environmental demands, some arising from physical environment and other from society. Some personality aspects help in better adjustment:

1. Showing strong motivation or commitment to some goal or outcome.
2. The most successful persons are somehow able to search for information needed to tackle the stress situation.
3. It has been seen that preplanning for future eventually help in better adjustment.
4. Distinguishing between that which can be changed and that which must be tolerated, taking whatever actions must be taken, make a major impact in adjustment.
5. Overall sustaining a mainly positive or hopeful rather than a negative outlook and an active engagement in the tasks of life over the long term.

Positive thinking and firm belief helps to build a good life adjustment. Life stress arises out of maladjusted behavior.

Emotion in health and illness

There are a range of emotions that individuals experience throughout day and night. Some of the emotions are significantly impart on health, illness and general well-being.

Anger: Anger is a collection of physical reactions, including particular facial grimaces and bodily positions characteristic of action in the autonomic nervous system particularly the sympathetic part. Anger may manifest like family-fury, outrage, resentment, wrath, irritability, hostility, violence, etc.

Physiological Changes: In anger, blood flows to the hands, heart rate increases, and a rush of hormones such as adrenaline generates a pulse of energy strong enough for vigorous action.

Fear: Fear is an emotional state in the presence or anticipation of a dangerous or noxious stimulus. Fear is usually categorized by an internal, subjective experience of extreme agitation, desire to flee or to attack and by a variety of sympathetic reactions of autonomous nervous system. Fear is often differentiated from anxiety on one (or both) of two grounds:

a. Fear is treated as involving specific objects or events while anxiety is regarded as a mere general emotional state.
b. Fear is a reaction to a present danger, anxiety to an anticipated or imagined one. While phobia includes an irrational, specific and persistent fear.

Physiological Changes: During fear, blood rushes to muscles, such as in legs, making the face cold and so on. At the same time, the body freezes, though only for a moment. Brain's emotional centers trigger a flood of hormones that put the body on general alert.

Sadness

One of the main functions of sadness is to help cope with significant loss.

For example: Death of a close relative. The individual generally withdraws from everything that in pleasurable or sociable. This creates the opportunity to mourn or loss or frustrated hope. Other feelings of sadness include grief, sorrow, gloom, melancholy, self pity, loneliness, dejection and depression, etc.

Love

Love is a pleasant emotion. Like love, tender feelings and sexual satisfaction involve the parasympathetic arousal. The related feelings of love may be family acceptance, friendliness, trust, kindness, affinity, devotion, adoration, infatuation, etc.

Psychological Changes: The parasympathetic action called as the 'relaxation response' is body wide set of reactions that generates a general state of calm and contentment, facilitating co-operation.

Happiness

Happiness is an enhanced activity in brain center that inhibits negative feelings and helps an increase in available energy and soothing of those that generate worrisome thought. This condition offers the body a general rest, as well as readiness and enthusiasm for whatever task in at hand and for striving towards a great variety of goals. The related feelings of happiness include family joy, relief bliss contentment, pride, delight, amusement, pleasure, thrill, gratification, satisfaction, euphoria, ecstasy, etc.

Physiological changes: In happiness, there is a general well being feeling which makes the body recover more quickly from the biological arousal of upsetting emotions.

Death, Dying, Bereavement and Loss

People initially react to challenging events by appraising the extent of the physical or psychological threat that they face and then assessing whether or not they have the resources available to cope. Anger, guilt, denial and sadness are normal emotions and usually transient in nature. However, the existence of such intense-feelings over a prolonged period is often an indication of psychological disorders and needs professional help.

Bereavement is a reaction occurring in response to the loss of someone or something very close to us. The expected loss of someone or something very close to us, the loss of a part of body or a loss of status are all threats to the self.

Physiological Changes: The fear of the unknown is often seen in the concerns of dying patients; who report that the possibility of losing control can cause greater anxiety than the thought of dying *per se* clients often fear being unable to control basic bodily functions such as elimination or fear of losing control of their mental functions or experiencing uncontrollable pain.

ALTERNATIONS IN EMOTIONS

Alternations in emotions are common. These occur due to various reasons. Unless the emotional reaction is upsetting normal efficiency in daily activities of the individual, not all kinds of alternations require medical attention:

1. Psychosomatic disorders occur when perceived stressors increase the susceptibility of the body to disease. This could bring with itself irritability and impatience in daily routine.
2. Temper tantrums are seen in children in the age of two and four, after which when they become shorter in duration and give way to throwing things in anger smashing doors and windows, sulking, etc.
3. Unexpected news, results, change in relationship status with friends or loved ones, undesired separation may also bring about alternations in emotions.
4. Illness, hunger, medicines, postoperative conditions may also bring alterations in emotions, which can be handled well by the individual itself.

Psychometric assessment of emtotions and attitudes

Theorists and psychologists try to assess an individual's evaluative orientations which will not only give us great insights into human behavior but also helps us to predict it:

1. Emotions can be assessed using emotional quotient test, also known as emotional intelligence rest (EQ). It is a standardized test which allows understanding oneself better and now days, employers who are using EQ test to select candidates for their recruitment, not just academically, for other disciplines also. Awareness of your emotional abilities allows you to improve your emotional intelligence and live a happier, more balanced lifestyle.
2. Emogram measures eleven basic emotions by presenting a series of photographs that precisely depict the emotions. Individuals respond to each photograph indicating a level of agreement with each photo. Different presenters are available to suit demographic needs. The basic 11 emotions that an emogram can measure are happiness, interest, surprise, contempt, disgust, anxiety, shame, fear, anger, distress and shame.
3. Attitude can be defined as a tendency to evaluate an object or event of a given class of stimuli in a positive or negative direction. Attitudes cannot be directly observed but are understood or inferred from external behavior, both verbal and non verbal. Attitudes have cognitive as well as emotional components. Very common attitude scales used are—Thurstone scale, likert scale, Bogardus Social Distance scale.

Chapter 6

Stress, Health and Coping

STRESS

The modern world lives under stress and strain. It has become a serious concern in present age. It takes a heavy toll on individual as well as nation's well being. It is a source for all aches and pains.

Stress can be defined as an internal state which can be caused by physical demands on the body or by environmental and social situations which are evaluated as potentially harmful, uncontrollable or exceeding out resources for coping.

Stress can also define as the pattern of responses an individual makes to events that disturb his or her equilibrium or exceed coping abilities. Stress also involves nonspecific physiological reactions that occur in response to stressful events, such as the increased flow of adrenaline that mobilizes us an extra effort.

Harry Gottesfeld defined stress as any interference, which disturbs the functioning of organism at any level and produces a situation natural for organism to avoid.

STRESSORS

The physical, environmental, social, economic causes of the stress state are called stressors. Physical diseases may be aggravated with stress and directly affect recovery. Stress is often a factor in cardiac problems. Now a days, stress management is a concern of health professionals:

1. Stress is one of the emotions that affect recovery directly. Chronic stress can lead to general wear and tear in the physiology of an individual.

2. Stress can impair immune system competence and pathological disease states or even death from exhaustion in very extreme cases.
3. The brain itself is susceptible to the long-term effects of sustained stress, including damage to the hippocampus and so to memory.

Kinds of Stressors

There are two kinds of stressors. One that cause distress and other as eustress. Distress occur when people experience unpleasant stressors, and those that cause eustress, which results from positive events that still make demands on a person to adapt or change. The newer definition of eustress includes the optimal amount of stress that people need to promote health and well-being.

Causes of Stress

Causes of stress are many and complex in nature. The following are the some of them:
1. Threats to self- concept or self- image and physical heath.
2. Situations involving conflict and ambiguity or vagueness.
3. Forced choices that have only unfavorable or undesired outcomes.
4. Novel events that lead the individual to believe that the situational demands will outstrip their ability to cope.

Stress Cycle

Stress can devastate the well- being of the body and mind in many ways. It has a number of immediate effects as well as long term effects. When stressors are maintained for a long time, behavioral, emotional and cognitive effects take place. If these effects continue to hamper the adaptation of the individual, there will be a cycle of distress. In other way, many people have learned to cope with stress well. This is called the wellness cycle. Educating people about adaptive ways of management of stress as to promote cycle is an important part of health professionals.

Distress cycle: The simplest way of explaining the distress cycle is to understand that, it is the stressors that create a feeling of overload on the individual's adaptive system. This stress overload, in turn, results in decreased output, mainly in productivity, enjoyment and intimacy.

Wellness cycle: It propagates that if health promoting lifestyle responses are made in reaction to the stressors, the individual learns to adapt better. This in turn ensures the overall benefits in terms of enhanced productivity, enjoyment and intimacy.

Post-traumatic stress disorder (PTSD): It is a severe stress reaction that is triggered by catastrophic events. It can have a lasting effect on individuals, leaving them a deep seated fear and a feeling that another traumatic event is waiting for around the corner (flash backs).

EFFECT OF STRESS

Psychologist Hans Selye (1956) was the founder of research concerning stress and its effects on human body. He studied the sequence of physiological reactions that the body goes through when adapting to a stressor. This sequence is called the general adaptation syndrome (GAS) and consists of three stages:

Stage 1. Alarm Reaction

When the body first reacts to a stressor, the sympathetic nervous system is activated. The adrenal glands release hormones that increase heart rate, blood pressure, and supply of blood sugar, resulting in a burst of energy. Reactions such as fever, nausea, and headache are seen in this stage.

During the initial alarm stage, the release of neurotransmitters epinephrine and nor epinephrine results in an increase in blood pressure and heart rate as the body is prepared for extraordinary levels of activity. Such high-level of arousal cannot be maintained however, and if the stressor is still present, the stress response moves into the second stage.

Stage 2. Resistance

During resistance stage, the high-levels of arousal that characterized the initial response are reduced to lower levels. But even these lower levels are above the normal level and stress hormones or corticosteroids are released as the body attempts to resist or combat the stressor. Even though the individual may no longer be aware that they are stressed, the body's reserve stores of fat and carbohydrates are slowly being depleted. The damage caused to the body's systems results in the emergence of diseases of adaptation, such as hypertension, eczema and diabetes.

Stage 3. Exhaustion

During the final stage, body's reserves are finally spent and the damage to the cardiovascular or immune system or any other system results in some conditions such as stroke, myocardial infraction, cancer or bacterial infection. Exhaustion can lead to stress-related disorder (SRD).

COGNITIVE THEORY OF STRESS

Cognitive appraisal theory of stress when proposed by Lazarus and Folkman in 1984. According to these theorists, individual's thinking about the stressor also contributes for the effect of stress. Lazarus and Folkman says that, stress occur only to the extent that the persons involved perceive (1) that the situation is somehow threatening to their important goals (primary appraisal) and (2) that they will be unable to cope with these dangers or demands (secondary appraisal).

Flow chart 6.1: Role of cognitive appraisals (Reference: Psychiatric Nursing Stuart)

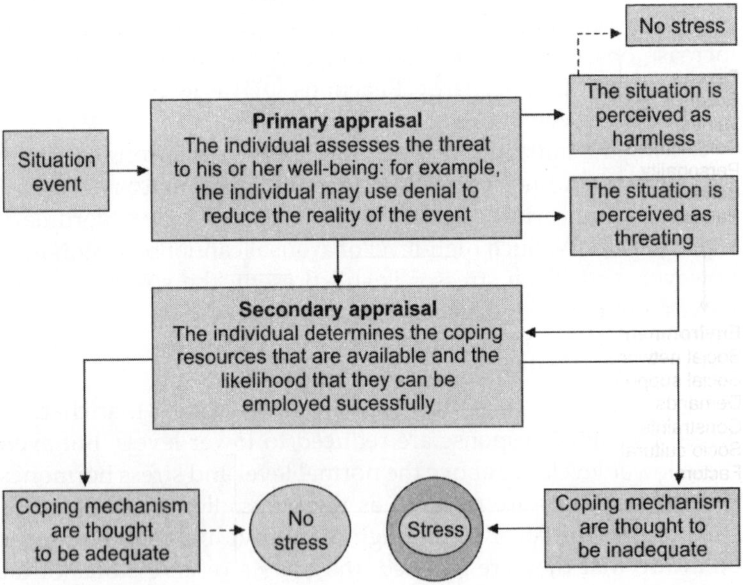

Adaptation to Stress and Coping

In 1984, Richard Lazarus published his classic work, stress, appraisal and coping. He argues that stress is much more complicated that stimulus response. He focuses on what happens inside a persons mind. He defines stress as a particular relationship between the person and the environment that is appraised by the person as taxing or exceeding his or her resources and endangering his or her well being. The experience of stress, the person's responses and the effects of stress are presented in the stress, coping and adaptation model. This system model has four components:

i. Antecedents to the stress
ii. Stress
iii. Coping and
iv. Adaptation

Adaptation Methods

Effective adjustment depends on how a person copes with anxiety or stress provoking situations of life. The coping strategies are

Flow chart 6.2: Stress, coping and adaptation model (Reference: Psychaiatric Nursing Stuart)

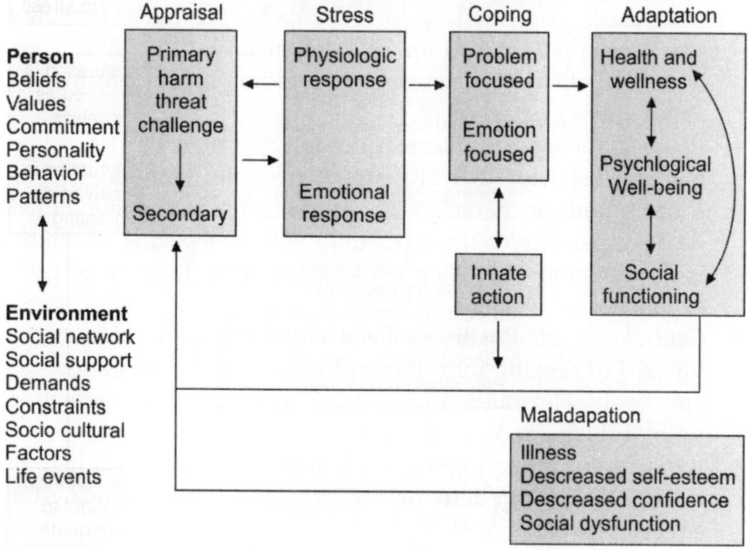

actions that people can take to master, tolerate or minimize the effects of stressors and they can include both behavioral and psychological strategies. There are two broad classes of coping:

1. Direct action
2. Palliation.

Direct action involves behavioral attempts to alter the troubled equation between a person and the environment in a number of ways. They include preparing toward a harmful agent, aggression toward a harmful agent and avoidance of that agent. Palliation is directed at reducing, eliminating or tolerating the distressing bodily, motor or emotional features of a stress emotion once it has been aroused by trouble in the environment. Taking palliative action means to soften or moderate distress, in short, to seek comfort, for example, by alcohol, drugs or use of defense mechanisms.

There are methods to cope with stress. Relaxation techniques, bio feedback, meditation, yoga, physical fitness regime, exercises, get-together, networking, time management and humor, etc. will help to reduce the stress:

- *Social support*: Social support may be in a variety of ways such as emotional support, self-esteem support tangible support, economic, network support. Emotional and self-esteem support may be offered by the nurse during periods when the client feels particularly depressed or low. Similarly, the nurse can offer tangible support in the form of practical advice and information that may help to relieve stress by providing health information about stress management.
- *Personal coping mechanism*: Coping style may be defined as habitual behavior that is a function of the individual's personality traits or characteristics. The extent to which individuals deal successfully or unsuccessfully with challenging situations is also determined by their personal coping style and their prior experiences and skills.
- *Control over self*: Positive belief about life helps to distress the life. Art of seeking information helps to deal with the person effectively. Flexibility and positive outlook regarding dealing with problems reduces the stress.
- Relieving or tolerating the some of the distress would help in better coping than denying the stressor and experiencing the effects later on.

- Maintaining a sense of self worth despite failures help in better adaptation.
- Better and harmonious relationships helps a person cope well despite being exposed to failure in life.
- Meeting the specific requirements of the stressful tasks that are being faced or utilizing the opportunities available for accomplishing any of the above, help to cope better.
- Joining humor clubs and has some fun: Play and humor makes the body and mind to relax. They help to prevent burnout.

ATTITUDES

Life is a mixture of likes and dislikes. How much we like or dislike something that colors our behavior. This behavior of like and dislikes can be termed as attitudes. Attitudes are simply expressions of how much we like or dislike various things. They represent our evaluations preferences toward a wide variety of attitude "objects". Our attitudes are based on information. For example, people who support the death penalty view it as a deterrent to crime and a just punishment. People who oppose it typically see the death penalty as a barbarian practice that does not deter crime.

Definitions

Triandis (1971)—An attitude can be defined as a tendency to respond positively or negatively, toward a certain idea, person or situation.

Kimball Yong—Defines, attitude as "a predisposition to respond, in a persistent and characteristic manner in reference to some situation, idea, value, material object or class of objects or person or group of persons". This can be a positive or a negative predisposition.

What Attitude Means

Actually, attitudes are the tendency to view life. This tendency of viewing is developed through people's experiences as they live with others and work, can affect the way they behave toward those ideas, people, objects, situation and can include opinions, beliefs and biases. In fact, attitudes influence the way people view these things before they have actually been exposed to them.

Attitudes are not inborn but they have learned through experiences and contact with others and even through direct instruction from parents, teachers, elders and other significant in a person's life. Attitudes involve a positive or negative evaluation of things, it's possible to go into a new situation, meet a new person or be exposed to a new idea with ones mind already made up to like-dislike, agree or disagree and so on.

The term 'attitude' includes several components, namely:

1. Cognitive, which suggests that attitude, is a consciously held belief or opinion.
2. Affective, which implies attitude, has an element of emotional tone or feeling.
3. Conative, which suggests the likely action as an outcome of the attitude.
4. Evaluative, which weighs the positive or negative aspects of the attitude.

The Nature of Attitudes

The prominent characteristic of attitudes is that they express anything in the form of evaluation. Evaluations are expressed in terms of dislike-like, pro-anti, favoring-not favoring, positive-negative, etc. Anything that arouses evaluative feelings qualifies as an object of attitudes. The object of attitudes can be:

- People (attitude toward self, others, friends, foes)
- Abstract concepts (attitude toward concepts such as domestic violence, single parenting, lesbianism and global warming)
- Entities (attitude about a teacher, a place, a movie).

Development of Attitudes

Development of attitude is the result of a number of different influences but learned phenomena. There are many reasons which may be instrumental in the development of attitudes. The basis for development of attitudes according to:

The ABC Model of Attitudes

This model of attitudes was proposed by Eagly and Chaiken in 1998. According to them, attitudes are made-up of three different parts. They are feelings, thoughts and actions.

Learning Theories

Attitudes can be formed simply by association. Instrumental conditioning, in which the reward consequences of any behavior shape its subsequent enactment, is directly relevant to development of attitudes, especially in social gatherings.

Consistency Theories

Consistency theories postulates that there is a tendency to maintain or restore balance in one's attitude structures. Any new attitude will be either accepted or rejected depending upon the fact whether it is consistent or not with the existing set of attitudes.

Cognitive Theories

According to cognitive theories, the person's cognitive organization plays the vital role in determining how information is interpreted, remembered or retrieved.

Group Memberships

The development of attitudes may depend upon the group membership that the person belongs to. For instance, if a person is campaigning for antidrinking behavior, he would have attitude in that direction conforming to his group behavior.

Existing Interpersonal Relationships

Development of attitudes also depend upon the existing interpersonal relationship between individuals. For insurance, there is a negative attitude against people of a particular religion, but at the same time if the individual is intimately involved with such a person belonging to that religion, this attitude many differ or vary from others.

Particular Situation

Though we say attitudes are more or less permanent there are situations where attitudes may vary depending upon the particular situation.

Factors Affecting Attitudes

Many factors affect in the development of attitudes are important as well as inclusive, when it comes to numbering the factors affecting attitude. Behavior can be influenced by a number of factors beyond attitude. These include:

1. *Preconceptions about self and others:* Preconception means the existing opinion or attitude about self, others or towards any object as such. This is one of the major factors affecting attitude, because it leaves little room for accurate judgment.
2. *Economic factors:* People who are economically sound may have different attitude towards different things than those who are not so sound.
   For example: Someone may have strong convictions about improving the public drainage system in their own town, but if it means a hefty increase to their property taxes, the economically backward people may vote against any improvements due to the potential for monetary loss.
3. *Social Influences:* The local social climate influences on the nature of attitudes.
   For example: An individual may be from very traditional background where wearing jeans is considered as an option. But when the individual joins with her companion in hostel away for home, she may opt to try it out.
4. *Convenience:* Attitudes are formed according to convenience of people which depends on place, time and accessibility of things.
   For example: Voting is necessary, but because of bad weather or if polling booth is too far from home, they may skip off.
5. Objects, people, events associated with pleasant experiences may take on favorable evaluations, while those associated with unpleasant experiences may be evaluated negatively.
6. *Kind of reinforcement:* Positive reinforced ideas becomes positive attitudes and those that are negatively reinforced taken on to form negative attitude.
   For example: A nurse who is noticed for regularity (positive reinforcement) for it would try to repeat her punctual timing.

BEHAVIOR AND ATTITUDES

Attitudes predict behavior. It predicts behavior under certain conditions especially when there is correspondence between (a) the measure of attitude and the behavior that is observed and (b) the presence of direct experience in the formation of attitude and the relevance of the attitude issue to the person whose behavior is being observed. In the absence of clear situational incentives and strongly held attitudes, people may deduce their attitude position by observing their own behavior.

For example: A student nurse is asked if she likes to serve sick and needy people, she may answer 'Yes' in affirmation because she may think she has chosen to study nursing, so she may be interested in this profession.

People hold complex views between attitudes and behavior that are further complicated by the social factors influencing both. Behaviors usually, but not always, reflect established beliefs and attitudes.

For example: People generally believe that they must take bath before worship and most people do so.

Unusually, positive attitudes manifest well-adjusted behaviors. However, in rare cases healthy attitudes may result in harmful behavior.

For example: Someone may remain in an abusive and potentially deadly domestic situation because they hold negative attitude towards divorce and breaking the relationship.

ATTITUDINAL CHANGE

The formation or change of attitudes is an ongoing process of living. There are three factors that contribute to attitude change.

1. The source
2. The message or content
3. The receiver.

For change in attitudes, it needs an impact, advertisers usually use celebrities to endorse products or to introduce concepts.

For example: A popular film heroin says that she is donating her eyes, which is a powerful way of sending a message for others to follow. Political figures are drained in advertisements for bringing children to polio booth for eradicating polio. These kinds of examples will help in understanding all the concepts that are very important in attitude change.

The Source

Message must originate from some source. It could be from a person, a group or an institution. The originator of the message is known as the source and various characteristics of the source affect the impact of the message. The source's credibility and attractiveness is particularly important.

a *Credibility:* It includes reliability and trust. If we have more reasons to believe a person, we are more likely to be persuaded by it. There are two main reasons for credibility. One is 'expertness' and the other is 'trustworthiness'. Expertness means special knowledge and skills. Trustworthiness is centered upon the truthfulness of the source.

b *Attractiveness:* Physical attractiveness are more likely to convince the people than those who are not.

The Message

The content of message is very important of persuasion and convincing:

a *Suggestion:* People may accept a belief from an attitude or be ready for an action by someone else's suggestion, without even requiring facts. Perhaps the most common form of suggestion is prestige or status based suggestion, in which the message appeals to people's regard for the sources status or prestige. Advertisers hire famous personalities for the very same reason.

b *Appeals to Fear:* The most common way of persuading people against some negative element is by making an appeal to fear. This is another method of making people change their attitude by scaring them.

 For example: The statement at crossroads says without helmet, it is "hell met" which goes to suggest that not wearing helmet could land you in hell. It has been held that appeals to fear work only up to a point. Strong appeals in fear, many backfire if people respond to them with a reaction called defensive avoidance. This means they avoid information putout by the communicator or refuse to accept the communicator's conclusions.

One-sided Versus Two-sided Messages

When it comes to attitude change, a one-sided approach is most effective when people are either neutral or already favorable to the message; a two sided approach is more likely to win people from an opposite point of view. A one-side approach is one in which the arguments are only the favor of the target object and a two-sided approach is one in which the message contains arguments in favor and also against the target object or issue in concern.

The Receiver

The person receiving the message may respond differently to the same content. The entire aspect of sending messages is to get receivers to do something they would otherwise not do. The study suggests that the characteristics of the receiver have a lot to do in understanding how much change may be there. They are:

a *Influenceability:* Generally, children are more persuaded than adults and also less educated people, illiterates are more easily influenced than the well educated.

b *Selective Attention and Interpretation:* Attitude change will depend on the factors like how much attention is given to a particular aspect and also how the message is interpreted. Selective attention means attending to a particular part and ignoring other parts of the message. We tend to avoid information which is very different to our own thoughts because it creates a difference known as discrepancy. Information that is very discrepant from our own position creates cognitive dissonance. Cognitive dissonance in an emotional state set up when two simultaneously held attitudes or cognitions are inconsistent.

c *Immunization:* According to Mc Guire, people resist counter messages to the extent that they have had a chance to rehearse their position. Mild exposure to arguments opposed to person's own position will immunize the individual against stronger attacks. This is similar to immunization to children against six killer diseases. Once the thoughts are immunized, change is difficult.

PSYCHOMETRIC ASSESSMENTS OF ATTITUDES

Attitudes vary in degrees. People vary on the strength of attitude. It can be measured. Attitudes can be measured by two methods.

1. Self-report methods
2. Behavioral measures.

Self-report Methods

Self-report methods are the methods where the scales or questionnaires are used to measure the attitude. A questionnaire tool consists of several questions related to one particular issue and in public opinion polls several attitudes are assessed with few questions from several people.

Attitude Scales

Attitude scales measure attitudes towards various things, people and concepts. For self-report measures, an attitude item consists of a question or statement about the object and a 'format' for the response. The format can be 'fixed', where the categories for the response are named or 'open minded' where respondents use their own words.

Involuntary Behavioral Measures

Involuntary behavioral measures are measured by some of the instruments.
For example: The galvanic skin response (GSR) which measures the electrical resistance of the skin. This resistance decreases when a person is emotionally aroused. The size of the pupil and facial muscles may also be indicator of arousal. The electromyography (EMG) recordings from the major facial muscles can indicate different emotions.

Attitude Scales

Attitude scales are framed with several questions or statements and every statement is graded with alternative answers like agree/ disagree, strongly agree/ neutral/ disagree/ strongly disagree. Every option is associated with weightage in numerical scores. Thus the subject answers every statement and numerical scores for all the statements are summed up to find out the strength of the attitude. The globally used attitude scales are:

1 *Thurstone's Scale:* It is a method of Equal – Appearing intervals. Thurstone (1931) developed this method. This method attempts to measure attitude on the basis of direct statements regarding the object of attitude. A large number of statements, both favorable and unfavorable are collected from various sources.

A	B	C	D	E	F	G	H	I	J	K	⟶

Unfavorable Neutral Favorable

'A' indicates the most unfavorable interval, 'K' represents the most favorable interval. The middle or neutral category is represented by 'F'. In all there are eleven cards on which A to K are written. Subjects will have to choose their responses from these cards. After the results of the entire sample are taken down the investigator will come to conclusion regarding the attitude in discussion; which can range from attitude towards any topic for example, live-in-relationship to religion conversion.

2 *Likert's Scale:* (Method of summated ratings). Likert in 1932 developed this scale to measure attitudes. In this type of scale, a large number of multiple choice statements usually with five alternatives such as strongly agree, agree, undecided, disagree, strongly disagree concerning the object of attitude are collected by the researcher and the results are tabulated together for final analysis.

For Example: Sex health education must be made compulsory in educational institutions.

Strongly agree	Agree	Undecided	Disagree	Strongly disagree
5	4	3	2	1

Guttman's Scale (Cumulative Scaling)

Guttman (1950) developed the cumulative scaling method. A large number of statements are collected regarding the object of attitude. Each statement has two alternative such as "agree – disagree" or more than two alternatives such as "agree, neutral and disagree". All these items are administered to a sample of hundred persons who respond to each item. All items are scored. On the basis of the total score, each subject is ranked from highest to lowest in terms of agreeability.

Bogardus's Social Distance Scale

It is a seven point scale consists of seven questions to the distance a person wants to keep in social set-up from other person belongs to some specific category. Every question is responded in yes or no questions are designed in such a manner that once the subject will say no it will be no to all the rest of questions. Numbers of no's tells the distance desired.

Nursing Applications

The nurse should have indepth knowledge regarding the development of attitudes. She should always keep in the mind that attitudes are learned phenomena and so they may be unlearned. Attitudes are prone to change. So nurse has to know that whatever behavior a person expresses at a certain point of time in his attitude position for that time and that it is not final. Patients sometime shows uncoperative behavior it may be as a result of lack of information. Health education helps to change their attitudes.

SUMMARY

- Motivation is an intrinsic phenomenon. It is purposive and need of the individual.
- Motives is a state of arousal that impels an organism to action. Motives are biopsychosocial in type.
- When goal is blocked, frustration arises. Conflicts give rise to frustration. Conflict resolution is an art and science.
- Emotions are the feelings of an individual. Feelings colors the life. It also affect health and illness.
- Any interference which disturbs the homeostasis of an organism is called stress. The causative factors are known as stressors. Stresses are biopsychosocial in origin. Adaptation to stress is called coping.
- Attitudes are the behavioral pattern of an individual to respond positively or negatively towards a certain idea, person or situation.

STUDY QUESTIONS

1. What is motivation? Explain the different theories of motivation.
2. What are motives? Describe various motives.
3. What is frustration? Describe of role nurse in conflict resolution.
4. Describe the development of emotions.
5. Enumerate different stressors and explain Seyles theory of stress.
6. What is an attitude? How does an attitude develop?

Chapter 7

Personality

PERSONALITY

The word personality has been derived from the Latin word "persona" which means a 'mask' that was used by actors on their faces while acting in drama. From this meaning it is clear that personality is synonymous with the outward appearance of an individual. It is considered as the uniqueness is one's character.

Personality Defined

According to Mark and Sherman—personality as "the characteristics pattern of behaviors, cognitions, and emotions which may be experienced by the individual and or manifest to others". GW Allport who defined personality as "the dynamic organization within the individual of those psychophysical systems which determine his unique adjustment to his environment.

In the words of Saundra K, personality is the unique way in which each individual thinks, acts and feels throughout life.

NATURE OF PERSONALITY

1. Personality is always dynamic and changing in nature. It is neither static nor rigid. It expresses and manifests itself differently in various circumstances.
2. It is constituted within the person. It develops in certain directions. It influences physical as well as our inner traits and life style.
3. Personality is a product of actions and their reactions. It is always active. It is never passive or static.

Types of Personality

Personality types are distinguished from personality traits, which come in different levels or degrees.

I. According to Hippocrates, four types of personality he identified.

I. Sanguine: It means the quality that is pleasant, cheerful. The person who is categorized as sanguine would be cheerful, vigorous and optimistic.
II. Melancholic: A melancholic person would be usually depressed, angry and easily irritable.
III. Choleric: A choleric type of person would be hot-tempered, angry and easily irritable.
IV. Phlegmatic: The person of phlegmatic personality would be slow-moving, calm and unexcitable.

II. Carl Jung, Classified personality into two types.

a. Introverts: These are reserved, thoughtful and self – reliant. They are not necessarily asocial, but they tend to have smaller circles of friends, and are less likely to thrive on making new contacts.

b. Extroverts: These are gregarious, assertive and generally seek out excitement.

Topography of Personality

Topography means detailed description a place or region. In psychology, Sigmund Freud, explained the topography of personality. According to him, mind consists of unconscious, preconscious and conscious parts. He compares these to iceberg. This is called the topographical model. Freud believed that the majority of what we experience in our lives, the underlying emotions, beliefs, feelings and impulses are not available to us at a conscious level. He thought that most of what drives us is buried in unconscious. Things that cause extreme anxiety are pushed down into unconscious. While buried there, they show their impact on us.

Freud also believed that everything we are aware of its stored in our conscious. At any some time, we are only aware of a very small part of what makes up our personality: most of what we are is buried and inaccessible.

Subconscious is in a half-way. We can access it if prompted, but is not in our active conscious. It's right below the surface, but still buried somewhat unless we search for it.

For example: Information such as cell phone number, best childhood memories etc. is stored in the preconscious.

The unconscious part is so large, and because, we are only aware of the very small conscious at any given time, this they have been linked to an iceberg, where the vast majority is buried beneath the water surface. The water by the way, would represent everything that but we are not aware of or have not been experienced and that has not been integrated into our personalities, referred as the nonconscious.

THEORIES OF PERSONALITY

Each theory of personality tries to define the word 'personality' in coherence with the theory. The most common theories of personality can grouped into the following:

a. Dynamic theories of personality
b. Type and trait theories of personality
c. Learning, and behavioral theories of personality
d. Humanistic theories of personality

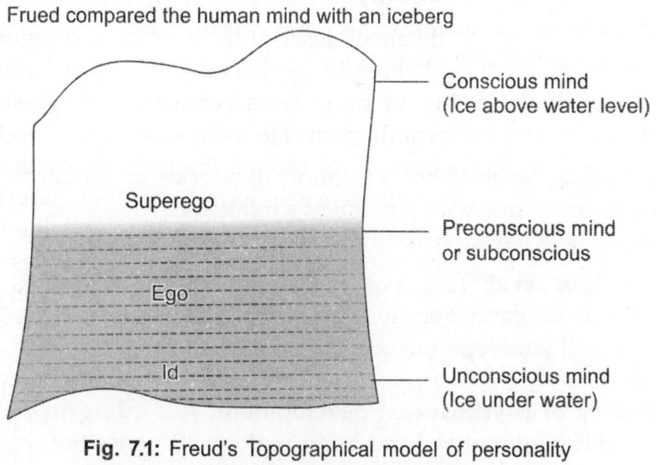

Fig. 7.1: Freud's Topographical model of personality
(Reference: Mental Health Nursing: Dr Bimla Kapur)

Dynamic Theories of Personality

Dynamic theories search for the processes by which needs, motives and impulses often hidden from view—interact to produce the individuals behavior.

Sigmund Freud's Theory of Psychoanalysis

Sigmund Freud's psychoanalysis is both a theory of personality as well as psychotherapy. Psychoanalytic theory has three major aspects:

a. A theory of structure of personality, in which the Id, ego and superego are the principal parts.

Id: It is the most primitive part and present in the infant. Id is a completely unconscious, arousal part of the personality that exists at birth, containing all of the basic biological drives. It operates according to pleasure principle.

Ego: The Id is managed by the ego. The ego consists of reality. It has the rules of behaving and thinking. The ego delays the satisfying Id motives and channels behavior into some more socially acceptable outlets by taking into account of what is possible in the real world.

Superego: It means over the self. It is fully 'conscience'. The superego consists mainly of prohibitions learned from parents and other authorities.

b. A theory of personality dynamics in which conscious, preconscious, unconscious motivation and ego-defense mechanism play a major role.

Conscious level: At this level, we are aware of certain phenomenona around us and of certain thoughts.

Preconscious level: Here, we found memories or thoughts that are easily available with a moment's reflection.
For example: What we had dinner at last night.

Unconscious level: This level contains memories, thoughts and motives which cannot easily call up. The entire Id is unconscious, the ego and superego include material at all three levels of consciousness.

c. **Theory of psychosexual development:** According to Freud, the different motives and body regions influence the child at different stages of growth. He believed that if a child's needs at one of psychosexual stages were either over satisfied or unsatisfied, fixation would takes places.

Oral stage: (Birth -1 year): In this stage, the infant obtains pleasure first by sucking and later by biting. Fixation at this stage many produce a critical, "biting" personality.

Anal stage: (1–3 years): Here toilet training takes place. It is the child's first interaction with authority.

Phallic stage: (3–5 years): Genitals are the main organs of focus.

Latency stage: (6-puberty): In this stage children grow and develop intellectually, physically and socially but not sexually. This is the age at which boys play with other boys girls play only with girls and each thinks opposite sex is pretty awful.

Genital stage: (Adolescence and beyond) Puberty marks the beginning when mature heterosexual interest appear.

II. **Jung theory of personality:** Carl Jung emphasized on people's future-oriented goals, hopes and plans. He credited each individual with collective unconscious and personal unconscious as an important aspect to understand an individual.

Collective Unconscious: It is believed to be part of the unconscious mind that went beyond the personal experiences of the individual. Collective unconscious grows out of the past experiences of the human race which is storehouse of primitive fundamental images, impression or predispositions. He called these images impressions or predispositions as archetypes. Archetypes are more like subjective recreations that originated in our ancestors in response to certain universal experiences—such as rising sun, rain and childbirth, etc.

Personal Unconscious: In addition to collective unconscious, each individual is credited with a personal unconscious, which develops whenever the individuals conscious experiences are repressed.

III. **Individual psychology of Adler:** Alfred Adler believed that people are forever struggling to overcome their feelings of inferiority. People strive continually for superiority and mastery of the world.

Inferiority complex: Adler believed that inferiority complex is the result of repeated failure to overcome weaknesses and inability to master or place excessive emphasis on some particular inferiority. He also stressed on the concepts of 'compensation' and 'over compensation' the pursuit of activities designed to make up for or to overcome inferiority.

Style of life: Adler also gave a term called 'Style of life' which each individuals own personal approach to living. Each of us develops a unique and lasting method of coping with life. This concept, along with the subjective nature of individual goals, led to the theory of Adler's individual psychology.

IV. **Interpersonal theory of Horney:** Karen Horney (1960) proposed that two major components of person, i.e. basic anxiety and basic hostility.

Basic anxiety: It is a feeling that arises in childhood when the child feels helpless in a threatening world. Loving and reliable parents can create a feeling of security, but erratic, indifferent or rejecting parents may increase the child's sense of helplessness and vulnerability. This sets the stage for basic anxiety.

Basic Hostility: It usually accompanies basic anxiety, because the hostility (negativity) cannot be expressed directly to parents, it is typically repressed, which only enhances the child's anxiety.

Horney also proposed three different modes of social behaviour. She believed that normal people use all three modes of social interaction at all times in a relatively balanced and flexible manner; adjusting their approach to situational demands. But disturbed neurotic individuals allow one approach to dominate their social interaction and this rigidity gets into trouble.

Moving towards others: This involves excessive compliance obeying.

Moving against others: This behaviour involves pursuit of satisfaction by dominating others.

Moving away from others: This is self protection by withdrawal.

V. Type and Trait Theories of Personality

Type Theory of Hippocrates

a. The Greek physician Hippocrates the father of medicine proposed his first type theory. The groupings or sets of types are called typologies. He grouped people into four temperament types:

Sanguine: Cheerful, vigorous, confidently optimistic.

Melancholic: Depressed, morose, gloomy.

Choleric: Hot-tempered, angry.

Phlegmatic: Slow-moving, calm and unexcitable

b. Kretschmer Theory of Personality: The German psychologist Kretschmer has divided people into four categories on the basis of their physical appearance and body built.

Pyknic: Short, fat and round. Show abnormal swings in mood, but generally popular and amiable persons.

Asthenic: Thin and simply built. Taller in comparison to their weight. Hands and legs are larger, muscles and bones not strongly built, breast undeveloped and short and the belly low and generally over sentimental.

Athletic: Neither much fat nor thin. Strong and well shaped. Norm in highest and handsome and healthy to look at. They have a balanced body and personality.

Dysplastic: These are the combination of above three. Generally, they like mental labor more than physical labor.

c. Sheldon Type Theory of Personality: Sheldon classified personality on the basis of physique in relation to their temperament as three types:

1. *Endomorph:* Simply, friendly, never crooked minded. They are lazy, slowy, sociable, sweep spearheaded and favor a good deal of entertainment.
2. *Mesomorph:* Well built and masculine. Dominating in nature. They do hardwork, happy and satisfied. Their mood, most of the time joyful.
3. *Ectomorph:* Weak and thin. Underdeveloped and under-nourished. Thoughtful and introvert. Like secrecy and never let others to know their thoughts.

d. Trait Theory of Allport: Gorden Allport described personality in three terms called:

Cardinal traits: These traits are dominating and influencing feature on the personality is such a way that it overshadows the influence of other traits in the same individual. These broad, highly influential traits are often called by names drawn from key historical figures.

For example: If you say someone is like, 'Jhansi Lakshmi Bai' it describes the cardinal trait of courage.

a. *Central Traits:* Central traits are those that might be mentioned in a careful letter of recommendation. These traits are not so prominent like cardinal traits;
   For example: Confident, reliable and punctual, etc.
b. *Secondary Traits:* These are the least generalized of the characteristics of the person. These are traits that are influential but only within a narrow range of situations.
   For example: Likes ice-cream, prefers movies would be description of secondary traits.

e. Rotter's Single-Trait Theory: Julian Rotter (1966) developed a questionnaire to measure internal versus external locus of control. "Locus of control" is the degree to which we believe that we cause or control, the events in our lives. If we believe that we are cause of most events, we have a highly internal locus of control. On the other hand, if we believe that most events are caused by luck, fate or powerful others, we have a highly external locus of control. We can learn useful things about a person by focusing on a single trait like locus of control.

f. Cattell's Trait Theory: According to Cattell the number of traits are many but most of them are found with each and every common person. Some traits are intrainsic and inherited, while some others originate from different situations. Other than these traits, Cattell professed surface traits and source traits:

1. *Surface Traits:* The traits which are clearly recognized and expressed in outer behaviors of an individual are called surface traits. Each of these traits includes many qualities of him and they work towards achieving the same goal.
   For example: A student showing proficiency in both mathematics and literature has a surface trait, because two different factors influence him to achieve success is these two subjects. Likewise some other surface traits are curiosity, honesty, unity, cunningness and dependency, etc.

Source traits: The inner qualities of human being which fuel behaviors and act as the source of surface traits are called as a source traits. Qualities like dominance, thinking, emotion, motivation, etc. are examples of source traits.

According to Cattell human personality develops being influenced by some active and forceful traits. In this process temperament supplies interest and enables the individual to undertake some sort of work. In every situation our temperament keeps us ready and active to do some work. Personality development is a complex process. It is influenced by both organic and environmental factors. So Cattell is of the view that personality is that human capacity which can change the reactions shown towards different environments.

g. Eyesenk's Classification of Personality: Hans J Eyesenk, a Germany psychologist proposed that personality consist of four dimensions. They are introversion, extroversion and normal mental deficiency. Later he added psychoticism as a new dimension

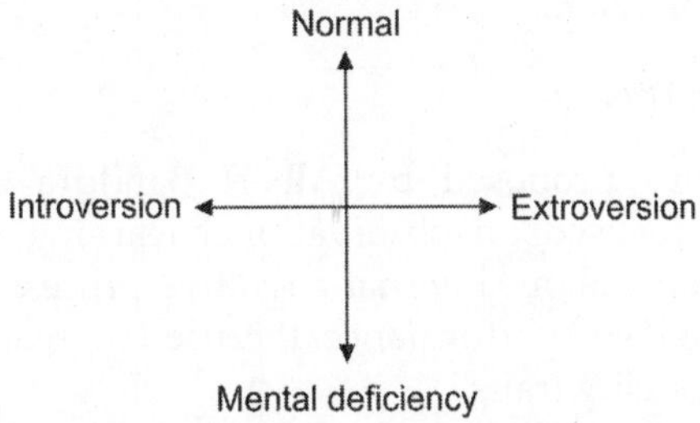

He observed that the person, who suffers from psychoticism is not fluent in speaking and can not adjust well to a new situation. His intention is not bold and his learning and memory power is not developed. This level of aspiration is also low. Psychotics suffer from mental disorders. They are quite different from introverts and extroverts. Persons suffering from mental deficiency are different from introverts and extroverts. They show different symptoms. In their case psychological factors are main and hereditary factors along with nerve diseases are subsidiary. On the other hand the man suffering from mental deficiency is dominatingly influenced by heredity and never sensations. After getting three dimensions of personality, Eyesenk accepted intelligence as the fourth dimension.

Learning and Behavioral Theories of Personality

According to learning and behavioral theorists, personality is a learned phenomenona. So it can be unlearned. Learning theorists seek to understand peoples behavior by studying their learning history, their current environment or both.

Dollard and Miller Theory of Social Learning

The basic idea behind these theories is that the behavior can be explained by means of basic learning principles derived from experiments.

Radical Behaviorism of Skinner/ Reinforcement Theory

According to BF Skinner, personality is actually a collection of reinforced responses. He placed strong emphasis on behavior that can be observed. The theory deals only with the processes by which reinforcement (reward) and punishment influence the likelihood of behaviors.

Social Learning Theory

This theory was proposed by Albert Bandura and Richard Walters. They focused on observational learning or imitation. They use concepts about internal cognitive processes to explain imitation and delayed performance. It is used to treat phobias and abnormal personality traits.

Humanistic Theory of Personality

Humanistic theorists emphasized on self concept of an individual. These theories are:

a. Roger's self theory: Carl Roger's self theory extracted from client-centered approach to psychotherapy and behavior change. As children grow, parents and others react to their behavior. Sometimes in a positive manner and sometimes with disapproval. He believed that in mature, adjusted people, there is matching (congruence) between the total person and the self. With this feeling, well adjusted people can accept the full range of their experiences without distorting or avoiding them. He coined the term called 'Phenomenal field'. It means the whole of experience. This is the individual's subjective frame of reference and it may or may not correspond to external reality. Out of the phenomenal field, a self or self – concept gradually develops.

MASLOW'S THEORY OF SELF-ACTUALIZATION

Abraham Maslow (1967) emphasized on the development of the self. According to him self-actualization is a goal that people are always striving to reach in life. These people live as a fully functioning person and fulfilled their basic potentialities.

Psychometric Assessment of Personality

The assessment of personality is to find out the thoughts feelings and behavior patterns. Personality can be assessed by variety of tests and methods. These are three types.

1. Subjective methods
2. Objective methods
3. Projective methods

Subjective Methods

These methods are in subjective in nature and involve the subjective reporting of the subject. These are as follows:

Interview

Interview is technique of assessment where the interviewer asks the questions for interviewee. It may be structured or unstructured. In structured interview the questions for the interview are framed in advance, but in unstructured interview, the questions are framed on the spot according to the need and demand. It has three phases: open, mid and close. Open phase includes rapport building. Next mid phase involves the questioning on the topic in focus. Both questions and answers are recorded. In last phase the interview will be winded up in an appropriate manner.

Interview has many drawbacks. It has less reliability and validity. It needs preparation and expertise.

Case History

In this method, indepth information about the subject is collected from his birth to present day. This helps to assess the personality of the subject.

Autobiography

Some people have the habit of noting down in diary every event of live and sometimes it may be given a book form. We can assess the personality by the writings.

Questionnaire

These are widely used tests in psychology. Questionnaires are developed which consists of various questions related to different traits of personally:

Various standardized questionnaires for assessment of personality are:

a. Eyescencks's personality inventory
b. Cattel's 16PF test of personality
c. Minnesota multiphase personality inventory
d. California psychological inventory

Objective Methods

In objective methods, assessment is made objectively so that the results should be reliable and valid.

Observation

In observation, trained people look the behavior in a controlled or uncontrolled way. The proceedings are recorded and analyzed. In this, variables of situation can be manipulated to see the effect of changes on the responses of subject. Recorded behaviors are analyzed and interpreted to know the personality of the subject.

BEHAVIORAL / SITUATIONAL TESTS

This test involves the presentation of an imaginary or hypothetical situation in front of the subject and he is asked to give possible reactions to the given situation. Sometime subject's possible reply is blocked with modification in situation and he is encouraged to give more replies.

For example: Subject is asked to imagine that you are at home alone and some antisocial elements enter your home what you will do? Let us assume that subject replies that he will ring to police for help. It can be blocked by modifying that suppose the phone is out of order. It this way every reply can be blocked to see the variety of replies subject can give. Subject's imagination of the mind and the kind of replies do help to assess the personality of the subject.

Rating Scales

Rating scales are helpful for the measurement about the different personality traits of a subject. Teachers, co-workers, parents, etc. can be asked to rate the subject for a particular personality trait. *For example:* Teachers are asked to rate the subject for his emotionality.

1	2	3	4	5
Manic	Excitable	Stable	Shy	Depressive

It is also called descriptive scale.
For example: A teacher can be asked to rate a student for his behavior in classes on the following rating scale.

1	2	3	4	5
Very good	Good	Average	Poor	Very poor

Maximum 1 to 5 or 1 to 7 digits can be allotted. Rating scales with numerical digits is called numerical scale.

Sociometry

Sociometry was founded by Moreno. It is mainly used to study the group and its relationship with others.

Projective Methods

According to Freud, projection is a defense or processes in which impulses, wishes and ideas are brought into conscious which were repressed in unconscious for being painful and embarrassing. Projection here is an unconscious process which bring out internal unconscious personality dispositions based in fears, desires and impluses. To externalize such unconscious personality tendencies subject is presented an unstructured stimulus. When the subject interpret and give meaning to it, his responses reflects his unconscious personality dispositions. These are the true reflection of the personality of a person. A trained psychotherapist interprets the type of personality.

Rorschach Inkblot Technique

Hermann Rorschach (1921) developed this test. There are ten inkblots, five in black ink on a white background and five in colored inks on a white background. These plates are standardized. Subject is presented these plates one by one and subject has to tell what he observes in these ink plates. He can give many response as he desires by observing from different angles to it. These responses are interpreted from various perspectives. The therapist assesses normal and abnormal personality traits by analyzing the information. This test is used to describe personality, diagnose psychological disorder, predict the type of behavior.

Thematic Apperception Test (TAT)

The psychologist Henry Murray and his colleagues in 1935 developed this test. In consists of 20 pictures, all black and white, that are shown to a client. Then, the client is asked to tell a story about the person or people in the picture, who are all deliberately drawn in ambiguous situations. Again, the story developed by the client is interpreted by the psychoanalyst, who looks for revealing statements and projection of the client's own problems onto the people in the pictures.

Three types of projective tests include the sentence completion tests, draw-a-person and house-tree person. In the sentence completion test, the client is given a series of sentence beginnings, such as "I wish my mother.." or almost everyday I feel….. and asked to finish the sentence, whereas in the draw-a-person and house-tree-person, the client is asked to draw the named items in detail.

Word Association Test

Word association test was developed by Jung. It consists of hundred words. Subject is instructed that he will be presented 100 words one by one and he has to respond immediately. Time is noted for response. The response is recorded. During this procedure, verbal and nonverbal responses are noted down. From these responses various complexes and sensitive areas of his life are identified and helps to understand his personality of the person.

Dream Analysis

According to Freud, dreams are the royal road to the unconscious mind. Dream contents do help to find out the various unconscious personality tendencies of the subject. Some contents are manifested in latent form. It shows the matter is most displayed in original way. It is required to interpret. Such latent content dream helps to undressed the personality of the individual.

Alterations In Personality

Personality traits are patterns of behavior that reflect how people perceive and relate to others and themselves. Personality disorders occur when these traits become rigid and maladaptive. A personality disorder is a problematic pattern occurring in two of the following four areas: cognition, affectivity: interpersonal-functioning and impulse control. A person with a personality disorder uses maladaptive behavior to relate to others and fulfill basic emotional needs:

1. *Antisocial Personality Disorders:* Person with antisocial personality disorder have a total disregard for the rights of others. They include 'psychopath' and 'sociopath'.
2. *Paranoid Personality Disorder:* The person with this disorder is having extreme distrust of others. The people will avoid relationships in which they are not in control or have the potential of losing control. They behave towards others with suspiciousness, envy, jealous and stubbornness.
3. *Obsessive Compulsive Personality Disorder:* It is characterized by a general psychological in inflexibility, rigid, conformity to rules and procedures, perfectionism, moral code and or excessive orderliness.
4. *Histrionic Personality Disorder:* The person with this disorder characterized by a pattern of excessive emotionality and attention seeking. These individuals are lively, dramatic, enthusiastic and flirtatious. They may be inappropriately sexually, provocative, express strong emotions with an impressionistic style and easily influenced by others.
5. *Schizotypal Personality Disorders:* It is characterized by a need for social isolation, odd behavior and thinking, and often unconventional beliefs such as being convinced of having extra sensory abilities.

6. *Depersonalization:* It is characterized by a detachment from one's sense of self and one's surroundings that leads to considerable distress and impairment yet an interact testing of reality. They have difficulty in perception, concentration and memory.
7. *Passive Aggressive Personality:* These people shows extensive inability to deal with interpersonal relationships.
8. *Borderline Personality Disorders*: It results in a pattern of instability in a person's mood, interpersonal relationship, self-esteem, self-identity, behavior and cognition. It is seen in childhood. Impulsiveness is its most prominent feature.
9. *Dependant Personality Order*: These people experiences an extreme need to be taken care of that leads to submissive, clinging behavior and fear of separation. It begins by early childhood, when behavior designed to elicit caring from others become predominant. These behaviors arise from the patient's perception that he is unable to function adequately without others.
10. *Neurotic Personality Disorder*: These are highly emotional and anxious in nature. During sickness, they react badly like excessive worried and tense and find difficulty in adjusting with their health and related problems. Less cooperative and highly anxious in certain factors.

PERSONALITY AND NURSING

Personality colors the life of an individual. So, it is the icon of health and illness. Personality and sickness are closely related. As a nurse, she should understand indepth about normal and abnormal personality traits. An indepth knowledge helps the nurse to predict the client's behavioral reactions in sickness and accordingly helps to develop suitable nursing strategies, keeping a good harmonious personality is a challenge to nurse and others.

SUMMARY

- Personality is the unique way individals think, feel and act. It includes character and temperament.
- The theories behind the personality are psychoanalytic, behaviorist, humanistic and trait theories.
- According to Freud, personality develops in a series of psychosexual stages, which includes oral anal phallic and latency.
- Jung developed a theory of collective consciousness.
- Behaviorists define personality as a set of learned responses or habits.
- Social cognitive view of personality includes the concept of reciprocal determinism, in which the environment, characteristics of the person, and the behavior itself all interact.
- Trait theorists describe the personality traits in order to predict behavior.
- Interviews, observation, scales, check-lists and rating scales are the method of measurement for personality.
- Use of personality knowledge helps the nurse to deliver a quality care.

TEST YOURSELF

1. What do you mean by personality? Explain with examples.
2. What are the types of personality?
3. Explain the topography of personality.
4. Enumerate the different measurement techniques of personality.
5. Explain objective method of assessment of personality.
6. Discuss the role of personality in health and illness.
7. Discuss the role of nurse in personality management.

Chapter 8

Developmental Psychology

The term development means a progressive series of changes that occur as a result of maturation and experience. It involves over all changes in the quality or character rather than in quantitative aspects. Developmental psychology studies the developmental changes covering the life span from conception to death. Life-span is divided into various stages which are associated with specific age periods. These are:

- The prenatal period (Conception to birth)
- Infancy (Birth – 2 years)
- Early childhood (2 – 6 years)
- Middle childhood (6 – 12 years)
- Adolescence (12 – 19 years)
- Early adulthood (19 – 40 years)
- Middle adulthood (40 – 60 years)
- Late adulthood/old age (60 and beyond).

PRENATAL STAGE

Prenatal stage includes from conception to birth. The nine months period is divided into three stages. These are the germinal period, the embryonic period and the fetal period. Family and maternal attitudes contributes for the relationship between mother and child during this period. Traditional beliefs and hazards affect the unborn child, maternal stress and unfavorable attitudes toward the child-to- be on the part of significant people.

The full term unborn or neonate has remarkable competencies to survive in the outside world. Many reflexes are well developed. Newborn are highly attentive to the wants around them. They look toward moving objects and listen closely to the sound of voices, especially their mother's voice, which they heard during inside the womb. These characteristics deepen parent's emotional attachments to their newborn.

INFANCY (BIRTH – 2 YEARS)

In infancy personality, social attachments, thinking and language first take shape. In this stage, the helpless newborn grown into a toddler with an impressive range of physical, cognitive, emotional and social skills.

Physical Development

During infancy, child makes considerable gains in height and weight, begins teething, develops sensory discrimination and begins to walk without support and talk.

Sensory acuity develops rapidly during the first three months of life. Child can capable of visual and auditory discrimination. After few days of birth, they react to loud noises, differentiates taste. Within three to four months, they can discriminate color and form.

Newborn can do motor movements, many of which are reflexive. Soon after birth, they can voluntary control of movements. They can crawl, creep and walk. Usually, walking starts by 13 to 15 months of age. Infants utter speech sounds, but retain only those heard frequently. By the end of first birthday, they can utter one and two word sentences.

Cognitive Development

By the time average infants have reached age of one year, triples its weight in the first two years, the brain is about 75 percent of its adult weight. By age five, the brain is at 90 percent of its adult weight. This increase makes possible a tremendous amount of major advances in cognitive development, including thinking, problem solving and memory.

After a few months of birth, infants can mentally group similar objects into a simple category; such as round, square, soft or flat.

Early in the first year, infants appreciate object permanence—the concept that objects and people continue to exist even when they cannot be seen.

Infancy is also when the basics of language development occur. At birth infants have a natural ability-surpassing that of adults to hear the differences between speech sounds in any of the languages even sounds they have never previously heard. They lose this capacity by the end of the first year, when their speech perception becomes specific to the language sounds they hear at home. The babbling becomes language specific. By the end of second birthday most toddlers combine words into simple phrases and sentences.
For example: "came, go".

SOCIAL AND EMOTIONAL DEVELOPMENT

Relationships between family members and care givers are vital for social growth of infant. Newborn pay special attention to faces and voices and social stimulation provokes greater interests and emotion than does interaction with others.

Infants exhibit many variety of expressing such a joy, distress, surprise, interest and sadness. These will be regulated by caregivers. In infants, emotional development in guided by parents and other significant members. As infants grow, they participate more with their parents in face-to-face play, i.e. mutual delight. By the end of first year infants have developed emotional attachments to their parents and rely on them for security and confidence, especially in unknown settings.

Secure and non secure attachments play a vital role in building confidence and trust. Secure attachments arise from sensitive, responsive care and provide a foundation of trust that an infant may generalize to other relationships. Insensitive or inconsistent care may instead cause infants to develop insecure attachments that are characterized by uncertainty and distrust in others.

Social, cordial relationships influence growth of self awareness and self-understanding. In the end of second year, toddlers become capable of self-recognition in a mirror and adopt other's evaluations of them when feeling proud or guilty.

EARLY CHILDHOOD STAGE (2 - 6 YEARS)

This stage is also known as infancy, in Latin it means "without speech". By two years child's thinking, remembering and understanding of emotion, self and social world revolutionizes quietly to a large extent.

PHYSICAL DEVELOPMENT

Height and weight of children enhances by 8 cm and add nearly 2 kg annually. Rapid physical changes are seen and body resembles those of adults. Because of continuous maturity, advances in memory, language and other abilities are refined and developed up to maturity level.

COGNITIVE DEVELOPMENT

Very eager to know the world. All the intellectual functions are working partially. In the case of memory, they recall very specific past experiences than all the happenings. Preschoolers are adept or solving practical problems. Most children lack logical reasoning skills that support formal or abstract problem solving.

For example: A five-year-old can figure out how nests are built? By the age five children master the basic principles of counting.

Language development is fast in this age period. By the age three, children are ready to make simple two or three word sentences and by six years, their vocabulary will be more than 10,000 words.

SOCIAL AND EMOTIONAL DEVELOPMENT

By the age of three-child's emotional repertoire include self-referential emotions such as pride, guilt, shame and embarrassment and the evaluations of others begin to influence the prescholar's self-concept. They show the signs of self-monitoring and motivation to be competent in performing skills. By the age three, child identify this own his/her.

The emotional attainment of young children to their parents and caregivers remain a cornerstone of physical well-being in early childhood. By as they develop their sense of self and learn to negotiate, compromise, resist and assert their own preferences and faces conflicts with caregivers. With the guidance of care givers preschoolers can better comprehend and empathize with other people's feelings and perspectives. This knowledge helps for coping in future.

MIDDLE CHILDHOOD PHASE (6 -12 YEARS)

In middle phase, children acquire enhanced capacities for judgment, reasoning, social understanding, emotion management and self awareness. At the same time, social circle widens and includes school, neighborhood, peer group and other influences. Children begin to perceive themselves in multiple roles and relationships besides family relationships.

PHYSICAL DEVELOPMENT

Children grow slowly and gradually in middle stage. They gain about 6 cm in height and 2 to 2.5 kg weight each year. Children especially become slimmer and body proportion change. Very well growth and coordination makes them to participate in sports and competitions.

COGNITIVE DEVELOPMENT

Schooling will fit in this age group. Children become capable of reasoning logically and systematically. Thinking also be more fluid and flexible. Children feel happy to master and enjoy their intellect and other cognitive skills like reading, mathematical ability, music and abstract thinking also improves. They are towards 'Learning by doing'.

SOCIAL AND EMOTIONAL DEVELOPMENT

Middle school children begin to develop a more complex, balanced self-image. They view on unique people and differentiate others in matters of skills and capabilities. Peer relationships and grouping takes place. They create small groups and try to maintain the cohesiveness of group. The social and cognitive advancements also provoke advances in moral development and altruistic behavior—behavior performed for the benefit of others without expectation of a reward. According to Kohlberg, children begin to perceive themselves as responsible to others because of the importance of getting along and of being a good citizen. They seek to act appropriately because people matter to them, not just to avoid punishment. Parents and community activities offer a sensitive ear and perceptive judgment.

ADOLESCENCE STAGE

Adolescence is the period from the beginning of the sexual maturity (puberty) to the completion of physical growth. It starts at about age 14 in males and 12 in females. It varies according to cultures.

PHYSICAL DEVELOPMENT

A hallmark of adolescence is a cluster of key changes at the primary sexual characteristics. Most notably, reproductive organs gradually increase in size. Along with changes in the primary sexual characteristics, boys and girls show changes in the secondary sexual characteristics.

For example: Body proportion, hair quality and distribution, voice and other physical features not directly related to reproduction.

COGNITIVE DEVELOPMENT

Abstract thinking and deductive logic develops. A general feature of formal operational thought is the ability to think in terms of the abstract concepts that link concrete objects or actions together.

SEXUAL DEVELOPMENT

Prepubescence leads to sex-drive. A new research show that 50 percent of adolescents under the age of 15 and 75 percent under the age 19 report having had sexual intercourse. It also showed that some adolescents are interested in or knowing about birth control methods and the signs and symptoms of sexually transmitted disease. So, illegitimate birth and incidence of STD's are increasing nowadays.

EMOTIONAL DEVELOPMENT

According to Hall, adolescence is a period of emotional stress, resulting from the rapid and extensive physiological changes occurring at pubescence. It is a period of "storm and stress," a time of heightened emotional tension resulting from the physical and glandular changes that are taking place.

EARLY ADULTHOOD STAGE

Early adulthood extends 19 years of age to approximately 40 years of age. It is a period of adjustment to new patterns of life and new expectations. The young adult is to play new roles in society such as spouse, parent and colleague.

PHYSICAL DEVELOPMENT

Physical changes in early adulthood are relatively minimal. The peak of physical health, sharp senses and mature cognitive abilities are seen around twenties, but even in this age group, signs of aging are already beginning. Oil glands in the neck and around the eyes begin to malfunction, contributing to wrinkles, in these areas near the end of the twenties and beginning of the thirties. The thirties may not bring noticeable changes, but vision and hearing loss starts by forties and fifties. In the forties, skin begins to show more wrinkles, hair turn gray or falls out, vision and hearing decline further and physical strength may begin to decline.

CONGNITIVE DEVELOPMENT

Biological intelligence achieves its optimum stage. Thinking and decision making ability improves with the experience of life and stability in life. Moral development and creativity show its superiority.

SOCIAL AND EMOTIONAL FAMILY DEVELOPMENT

In this period, making a family, fully, relations and work life starts. Network of social contacts develop and spread fast. Work area "stress plays the role in this age of life".

MIDDLE ADULTHOOD STAGE

PHYSICAL DEVELOPMENT

In the fifties, physical changes are noticeable. The performance of major organ systems too decline. Throughout middle age, weight may increase as the rate at which the body function slows down but eating increases and less time is spent on exercising. Height begins to decrease, with about half an inch of height lost of every 10 years past age forty. The most dramatic change is climacteric. Change in sexual functioning of the reproductive system and various aspects of sexual activity change greatly. Female experiences menopause and males may experience less production of semen. In male prostate gland also get enlarged, which not only interfere with sexual activity but also with urination.

COGNITIVE DEVELOPMENT

Changes in memory storing and processing is seen. Biological intelligence remains constant with a slight decline in it. Moral development reaches its peak and the individual take time for decision making. It is a period of creativity.

SOCIAL AND EMOTIONAL DEVELOPMENT

Social network will reduce and lasts for long life. Increasing age, retirement and physical health conditions limit the social life. Emotionally, old people do share their emotions of joy and happiness more frequently but share sad and negative experiences and feelings less frequently.

LATE ADULTHOOD/OLD AGE (60 YEARS – DEATH)

PHYSICAL DEVELOPMENT

Ageing is a natural phenomena. Physical decline takes place globally and depends on prior health illness conditions and cultural contributions. Natural aging is called primary ageing and ageing because of disease or abuse of the body contributes for secondary aging. Primary aging changes seen in all the systems of the body; like vision, hearing, smell, taste and other senses. Slowing of reflexes and response time enhances with respect of age.

COGNITIVE DEVELOPMENT

Decline in memory, i.e. amnesia is observed in later life period. Episodic memory is more affected than long term memory. Degeneration of brain cells or declining health conditions contributes for memory loss. Memory disorder like Alzheimer's disease is the result of aging.

SOCIAL AND EMOTIONAL DEVELOPMENT

Social circle will be very narrowed because of death of friends, poor health conditions and departure of friends with personal factors. loneliness and fear of death results in psychological disorder like depression and anxiety. Emotional control is high and control on emotional expression is high. But, it does vary from individual to individual.

VULNERABLE GROUPS AND CHALLENGES

There are certain group of people who are more vulnerable than others in all matters involving physical, social or psychological hazards.

For example: Sick, women, children, old aged people and physically and mentally challenged persons.

SICK PEOPLE

Sick role includes inhibition of normal social behavior.

In Childhood: Because of immaturity in different systems and immunity gives rise to sickness. If normal development will not occur in this period, children will be fixated and shows disorders in future life.

Sometimes sickness in childhood may be real or pseudo. If home discipline is relaxed, children try to receive more attention than usual. As a result of this, they may show conversion like symptoms and tries to avoid an unpleasant task or situation.

In old age: Many older people suffer from imaginary illness and concentrate on any pain or ache and exaggerate it out of proportion. Sometimes they may suffer from genuine sickness. While some learn to cope with their physical aliments and some may fail and visits doctors often.

CHALLENGED PEOPLE

Challenged people either physically or mentally challenged. Providing care and rehabilitating them is corner stone of every health personnel and citizen. Many physically challenged people do not like help being offered to them unless they themselves ask for it; because of self-respect. Coping with themselves and others plays very important role. Empathetic care helps them to do well in social life.

WOMEN

Women who lost their husbands or divorcee pose major adjustment problems in life. They have to face their own life and as well as social life. Working woman too adjust in office as well as at house also. This requires readjustment. Proper management techniques helps to overcome the burnout at different levels.

PSYCHOLOGY OF GROUPS

Man is a social animal. Form birth to last breath, he lives in society. A social group is a basic social unit when two or more persons interacting with each other, interrelationships are directed towards fulfillment of certain common goals or purposes. Inter stimulation and response are the key factors in the process of social interaction. Group shares a common identity and goal. Different members of a group may have different purpose to be in the group but they share cooperation and coordinate in such a manner that whole group moves toward a particular goal. In infancy, groups are not formed. When child attains school age, group behavior emerges. It is exhibited as group play. In adolescence, group behavior becomes more powerful and in adult life, it booms to large extent. By living in a group, individual grows and finds success in life. Most of the activities in adulthood done by groups. Success of life is achieved by coordination and harmony of the group members. Better understanding and interpersonal relationships in group members promotes better a sense of we—feeling and well-being.

CHAPTER SUMMARY

Development means a progressive series of changes that occur as a result of maturation and experience.

PRENATAL DEVELOPMENT

- It includes from conception to birth.
- Dominant genes control the expression of trait, whereas recessive gene traits are only expressed when paired with another recessive gene for the same trait.
- The fertilized egg cell is called a zygote and divides into many cells, eventually forming the baby.

POSTNATAL DEVELOPMENT

- Four critical areas of adjustment for the newborn are respiration, digestion, circulation and temperature regulation.
- At birth, infant's reflexes include sucking, rooting, motor, grasping and babinski. Vision is blurry and lacking in full color perception until about six months of age. Gross and fine motor skills develop at a fast pace during infancy and early childhood.
- Piaget's stages include the sensorimotor stage of sensory and physical interaction with the world, preoperational thought in which language becomes a tool of exploration concrete operations in which logical thought becomes possible, and formal operations in which abstract concepts are understood and hypothetical thinking develops.
- The stages of language development are cooing, babbling, one-word speech and telegraphic speech.
- The three basic infant temperaments are easy, difficult and slow to warm up.
- The four types of attachment are secure, avoidant, ambivalent and disorganized – disoriented.

ADOLESCENCE

- Adolescence is the period of life from about age 13 to the early twenties during which physical development reaches compelition.
- Puberty is a period in which the sexual organs and systems fully mature and during which secondary sex characteristics such as body hair, breasts, menstruation, deepening voices and the growth spurt occur.
- In Erikson identity versus role confusion crisis the job of the adolescent is to achieve a consistent sense of self from among all the roles, values and futures open to him or her.

ADULTHOOD

- It begins in the early twenties and ends with death in old age. It can be divided into early or young adulthood, middle adulthood and late adulthood.

- The twenties are the peak of physical health: in the thirties the signs of ageing become more visible and in the forties vision problems may occur, weight may increase, strength may decrease and height begins to decrease.
- Women experience a physical decline in the reproduction system called the climacteric, ending at about age 50 with menopause, when a woman's estrogen levels are at zero and her reproductive capabilities are at an end. Man goes through andropause, less dramatic changes in testosterone and other male hormones, beginning in the mid twenties.
- Reaction time slow down, but intelligence and memory remain relatively stable.
- Eriksson's crisis of young adulthood is intimacy versus isolation in which the young person must establish an intimate relationship, usually with a mate.
- The crisis of middle adulthood is generativity versus stagnation, in which the task of the middle aged adult is to help the next generation through its crises, either by parenting mentoring or a career that leaves some legacy to the next generation.
- Erikson's final crisis is integrity versus despair in which an older adult must come to terms with mortality.
- The five stages of reaction to death a dying are anger, bargaining, depression and acceptance.
- Two or more individuals who have common objects and shares similar feelings and attitudes is called group. Groups are formed in short age period and becomes very significant and strong in later years of life.

REVIEW QUESTIONS

1. What physical changes occur during puberty?
2. According to Erickson, what is the most important crisis faced by adolescents?
3. What physical, psychological and emotional changes occur during early and middle adulthood?
4. What do you mean by vulnerable group? Explain any one in detail.
5. Define group. Explain the group behavior.

Chapter 9

Mental Health and Mental Hygiene

CONCEPTS

In this new millennium, life has become more materialistic, mechanical and moreover very stressful. People's needs are multiplying and competitiveness has increased a lot to combat daily life. As a result of this life style, human is suffering not only with physiological disorder but also with the problems of mental health.

The World Health Organization (WHO) defines 'health' as "a state of complete physical, mental and social well-being and not merely the absence of disease or infirmity".

According to Dunn (1961) describes that people are not simply ill or well but their degree of health changes according to their inner or outer circumstances. Inner circumstances refer to human biology. Outer circumstance includes environmental factors. So, health of an individual changes according to bodily factors, situational and environmental factors.

Mental health is a concept that refers to a human individual's emotional and psychological well-being. Webster defines mental health as "a state of emotional and psychological well-being in which an individual is able to use his or her cognitive and emotional capabilities, function in society, to meet the ordinary demands of everyday life".

To say a man has good mental health, it describes how he/she effectively and successfully functions in society. Feeling comfortable, happy, capable and competent, being successfully to handle normal levels of stress, maintain satisfying relationships and lead an independent life and being able to "bounce back" or recover from difficult situations, are all signs of mental health. From this, we can state that mental health as a continuum. It varies according to one's philosophy, values and attitudes.

Mental hygiene is a way of life to maintain mental health. Maintenance of normal mental hygiene signifies harmonious adjustment to himself and environment. It is greatly affected by poor frustration and conflict management. It is a part of health psychology. Health psychology studies the relation between psychological variables and health, reflects the view both mind and body are important determinants of health and illness. Health psychology believes that our beliefs, attitudes, and behavior contribute significantly to the onset or prevention of illness.

Mental Hygiene Defined

Mental hygiene is a means of achieving mental health. Let us consider some of the definitions of mental hygiene which will help us to understand its nature and functions.

- HW Bernard, "mental hygiene is simply the means by which the process of mental health is realized…. mental hygiene is a way of life and so involves all that influences what one feels, says and does".
- DB Klein defines "mental hygiene is concerned with the realization and maintenance of the minds health and efficiency".
- JA Hadfield, "mental hygiene is concerned with the maintenance of the mental health and the prevention of mental disorders".
- CV Good, "In its broadest sense, the aim of mental hygiene is to help all persons achieve fuller, happier, more harmonious and more effective lives".
- English and English – defines 'mental hygiene is the study of principles and practice in the promotion of mental health and the prevention of mental disorder".

Mental Health and Mental Hygiene

In this manner, mental hygiene is a manner of life in which the individual's adjustment to his environment is maintained intact.

According to NE Cutts and N Moseley, mental health is that ability by means of which we establish our adjustment with the different situations. Life and mental hygiene is that means or tool which makes this adjustment possible. Mental health is the end and mental hygiene the means.

Characteristics of Mentally Healthy Person

Mental health is often said to be a state of well-being associated with happiness, contentment, satisfaction, achievement, optimism or hope. These terms are difficult to define and their meanings change as they relate to a particular person and life situation.

Some theorists have suggested that mental health cannot be confined to a simple concept or a single aspect of behavior. Instead, it incorporates a number of criteria that exist on a continuum with grades or degrees. These criteria form the basis of the optimum of mental health. However, they are not absolute, and each person has limits. Although no one reaches the ideal of all the criteria, most people can approach the optimum.

Criteria of Mental Health

The following six criteria are indicators of mental health:

1. Positive attitude toward self
2. Growth, development and self-actualization
3. Integration
4. Autonomy
5. Reality perception
6. Environmental mastery.

1. Positive attitudes toward self include an acceptance of self and self-awareness.
2. Growth, development, and self-actualization mean that the individual seeks new experiences to move fully explore aspects of oneself.
3. Integration is a balance between what is expressed and what is repressed, between outer and inner conflicts.
4. Autonomy involves self-determination, a balance between dependence and independence and acceptance of the consequences of one's actions.
5. Reality perception is the individual's ability to test assumptions about the world by empirical thought.

6. Environmental mastery enables a mentally healthy person to feel success in an approved role in society.

Characteristics of Mentally Healthy Person

Mental wellness is generally viewed as a positive attribute, such that a person can reach enhanced levels of mental health, even if they do have any diagnosable mental health condition. This definition of mental health highlights emotional well-being, and the capacity to live a full and creative life; as well as the flexibility to deal with life's inevitable challenges. According to Meyer, Sweeny and Witmer's Wellness model, it includes five life tasks essence or spirituality, work and leisure, friendship, love and self-direction and twelve sub tasks, sense of worth, sense of control, realistic beliefs, emotional awareness and coping, problem-solving and creativity, sense of humor, nutrition, exercise, self-care, stress management, gender identity and cultural identity are identified as characteristics of healthy functioning and a major component of wellness. These components provide a means of responding to the circumstances of life in a manner that promotes healthy functioning.

Another way of summing up the characteristics of a mentally healthy person can be as following:

1. An optimal perception of reality: The mentally normal individual is usually realistic in his appraisal of his own reactions and abilities. He knows that what is going on around him and perceives as it is.

2. Knowledge about self: The normal healthy person knows his own feelings or behavior and he is accountable for it. This lacks in mentally-ill person.

3. Adjustability: Mentally healthy person can also adjust well in the complicated and complex situations of life. He is capable of achieving the goal and solving the problem without effecting his surroundings. He handles the situation being calm and with patience so that other people should feel happy.

4. Self-confidence: A healthy individual is always feel self-confident. He never looses aspiration in stressful situation. He faces the complexities of life with confidence with an aim to be victorious in these conditions.

5. Selection of life goal: A mentally healthy person chooses the goal in an accurate and in a realistic way, and strives to achieve it.

6. Emotional stability: A mentally healthy individual exhibits emotional control and stability according to the need and demand of situation.

7. Sexual maturity: A mentally healthy person satisfies his sexual needs within the socially approved ways and sources.

8. Satisfaction in accomplishing tasks: A mentally healthy person not only take every task with sincerity and honestly but also feel satisfaction in working and accomplishing the taken task. He always feel pleasure in doing the work.

9. Absence of extremism: A mentally healthy person lacks extremism in his desires and wishes. He does not desire for excessive money, respect, honor, etc. His desires and wishes are retained within moderate limits.

10. Productivity in using one's abilities: A mentally healthy person is able to use his abilities whether less or more in productive activity. He has certain enthusiasm for living and does not have to drive himself to meet the demands of the day.

11. An ability to form affectionate relationship: A normal healthy individual is able to form close and satisfying relationships with himself and with other people. He is sensitive to others needs and feelings and does not make excessive demands for the gratification of his own needs.

12. Regular life: A mentally healthy person lives on a defined time table. His work, interaction, and other activities are regular and according to the values and beliefs of society and culture.

Warning Signs of Poor Mental Health

1. Inefficient perception of reality: The individual does not evaluate his capabilities in a fairly realistic manner. Either he over evaluates his abilities or he tries to tackle more than he can accomplish. He may shy away from a difficult task because he underestimates when he can do.

2. Lack of self knowledge: The person may try to hide important feelings and motives from himself. This makes him poorly informed of his own true likes and dislikes and his personality will start showing conflicts.

3. Inability to exercise voluntary control over behavior especially of sexual and aggressive nature.

4. Low self-esteem and in-acceptance: He always feels obligated to give in to others opinions when dealing in a group. Feelings of worthlessness, alienation and a lack of acceptance by others are prevalent among mentally ill clients.

5. Usually the person is so concerned with protecting his own security that he becomes extremely self-centered; he is preoccupied with his own feelings and strivings and can only seek affection, without being able to reciprocate.

6. Unproductivity: The person lacks enthusiasm for living and has to drive hard to meet the demands of the day. He also lacks energy and has excessive susceptibility to fatigue.

Promotive and Preventive Mental Health Strategies and Services

The current trend in mental health practice is on preventative and promotive services at institutional and community settings. A number of strategies are adopted to promote mental health and prevent mental health from the hazards of illness. The strategies can be broadly discussed as:

1. Mental health education: Education plays the most important part in illness prevention, as many people do not recognize the risk to illness present in their lives. Or they are unable to implement the knowledge that they have owing to the pressures of their everyday existence.
For example: Anti-drug use campaigns. Those least able to afford tobacco/ alcohol/ other addictives consume them the most. Through, education to health personnel in turn to the community in the form of health talk, drama, exhibition and mass media helps to reduce the incidence of psychological disorders.

2. Habits and life style: Use of drugs, alcohol, smoking, irregular exercise, etc. contributes for the formation of physio-psychological disorders. Educating the community on the aspects of healthy habits and life style management reduces the incidence of psychological diseases.

3. Adherence to psychiatric follow-up: Proper compliance to medications and medical treatment helps to reduce the prevalence of diseases. Use of community health nurses, NGO's, local health personnel and networking contributes a lot in psychiatric rehabilitation and also helps to reduce residual symptoms.

4. Guidance and counseling: Psychotherapy is the treatment of behavior disorders by psychological means. It requires therapists who have full knowledge about its application. Nurses, can provide guidance according to the requirement of clients. Many a times, people who have given up drug addiction have been used to guide and counsel (e.g. Alcoholic anonymous) to other drug addicts. So, guidance and counseling when dealt by experienced hands provides better results.

5. Psychosocial rehabilitation: Involvement in useful work or being employed on the basis of competitiveness, keep individuals in touch with reality and enhances self-esteem, provided that they accept the work as dignified and suited to their abilities and interests.

6. Social participation: Involvement in social activities make people feel less isolated and more related to others. Since the circumstances of the modern day life tend to produce more loneliness, social participation of any kind provides for the right emotional development that promotes mental health.

7. Self-understanding: People can improve their mental health through self-understanding. A person who learns to accept his feelings as something natural and normal has adjustment with the realities of life than a person who lives under some kind of denial. Also by discovering the occasions that provoke emotional overreaction, person can learn to guard against it.

EGO-Defence Mechanisms

'Ego' means 'reality'. According to Sigmund Freud, the ego disguises, redirects, hides and copes with the Id's urges. Ego defense mechanism are those mechanisms by which our reality is guarded (defended) and at the same time implemented by translating our real motives into something that we can handle. The defense mechanisms are generally accepted way of looking at how people handle stressful situations and conflicts. They are used as a way of coping.

Defense mechanisms or mental processes are at unconscious level. They are used to reduce anxiety or resolve conflict. Conflict tends to arise when a person has to resolve two equally strong opposing impulses or desires, e.g. a student has to attend the class, whereas at the same time, she has to attend a marriage function.

There are two opposing desires which she is finding difficult to resolve. The conflict then leads to increased anxiety. To overcome this anxiety a person's behavior is direct to reduce this threat. This mechanism of self-protection is known as defense mechanisms or mental mechanisms. Some of the very common defense mechanism are:

1. Compensation: People, who do not possess certain skills, happen to have some other qualities, or skills that overwhelm their inability. The lack of something is hidden by having a more prominent feature of the personality that compensates or makes up for their inability.

For example: People who may not be very good in socializing skills may be very good in singing or dancing. This will get them enough attention which they would have missed otherwise for their lack of socializing skills.

The origin of this defense mechanism can be seen in the infant who substitutes his thumb or a toy for the nipple of the bottle in order to relieve tension and make up for some of the pleasurable sensations of sucking that the infant may be lacking in sufficient quantity.

2. Denial: In order not to face the unpleasant situation, the individual altogether denies the reality. A person instead of learning to accept the reality as something natural and normal tries to escape them by denial.

For example: An alcoholic denies the amount he consumed.

3. Displacement: In this defense mechanism an emotional feeling is transferred to person or objects who are less dangerous than those who initially aroused the emotion.

For example: Father blasts the child for not doing well in test. The child gets angry but cannot shout back at father. So he starts quarrelling with his brother or sister. It shows that he is displacing his anger from father to his brother or sister.

4. Fixation: It refers to the point in an individual's development at which certain aspects of the emotional development do not advance and fixated at that stage. This arrest appears to develop from the inability of the individual to solve problems that occurred during the specific phase of development at which progress ceased or stopped.

For example: Alcoholics are believed to be fixated at the oral stage of development.

5. Repression: Repression represents those memories, feelings and thoughts that are stored in the unconscious because their recall may be painful or fearful. Much of what is repressed occurs in childhood and therefore may not be readily verbalized. Because repression is usually limited to specific areas or topics. Repression operates wholly on an unconscious level. Unacceptable feelings are unconsciously kept out of awareness.

For example: A man is jealous of his good friend's success but he is aware of his feelings of jealousy.

6. Rationalization: It is a commonly practiced defense mechanism that seeks to justify or provide a seemingly reasonable explanation to make undesirable or questionable behaviors appear logical, reasonable, or acceptable. It is frequently used to modify guilt feelings because the valid or true explanation for the behavior would produce feelings of guilt or anxiety. A phrase 'grapes are sour' is an example of rationalization.

7. Regression: The return to an earlier form of behavior or stage of development is called regression. This usually occurs when the more mature or appropriate behavior is blocked by feelings of uncertainty, anxiety, fear, conflict or lack of reward. In some instances, it will also represent a retreat to earlier responses. Sometimes an adult throws temper tantrums and tears is an example for regression.

8. Identification: Identification gives one satisfaction or compensation by identifying with others and their achievements. In identification with others, an individual may actually acquire new and useful behaviors.

For example: After hospitalization for a minor surgery a girl decides to become a nurse because she developed a desirable attitude found in people whom she respects and admires.

9. Over compensation/ Reaction formation: Reaction formation is the display of behaviors as attitudes that represent the opposite of one's repressed feelings. Anxiety and guilt feelings are repressed and their opposites expressed instead.

For example: A woman who actually dislikes her mother-in-law hides her feelings by being always very nice to her.

10. Substitution: Substitution may be employed to reduce tension resulting from frustration. To get satisfaction and reduce anxiety, resulting from frustration the substitutive action must have certain similarities to the frustrated one.

For example: A student who has not got admission to medical, try to institute it with a course of nursing.

11. Conversion: In this mental mechanism, the strong emotional conflicts are expressed as or converted into physical ailments. It operates wholly on an unconscious level.

For example: The boy who hates father and likes to strike at him, if he does so develops a paralyzed arm. The conflict is resolved. He cannot strike his father even if he wishes to, and the situation carries no threat of retaliation.

12. Introjection: In introjection the values and characteristics of significant persons are incorporated in one's personality. For instance, a woman who like to live in a simple way introjects in her the sophisticated way, of living like her husband.

13. Transference: In transference, the image of one person is unconsciously identified with that of another. A patient who is fond of his daughter finds the nurse of the same age and height as his daughter. So he transfers his positive emotions to his nurse as his daughter. It is also possible that if he dislikes his daughter he transfers his negative emotions to the nurse by being rude, abusive or aggressive without any cause.

14. Suppression: Suppression is a conscious effort is made by the individual to dismiss the impulses, feelings and thought that are unpleasant to the preconscious mind. So unacceptable feelings and thought are consciously kept out of awareness.

For example: A student taking an examination is upset about an argument with his friend but puts it out of his mind so that he can finish the test.

15. Sublimation: It is a positive mechanism. It consists of a redirection of sexual impulses to socially valued and accepted activities. Unacceptable desires find an acceptable outlet.

16. Projection: Projection means blaming others as a way of coping with one's unwanted motives by shifting them to someone else. A student who wants to skip classes may project that everyone is skipping classes and hence, it is okay. But in reality, others may not be skipping classes. If projection is overused, it may give rise to a behavior disorder called paranoia. People with this disorder may translate their own negative feelings onto others; and feel that others are out there to get them humiliated or even killed.

17. Sympathism: The individual in sympathism tends to always seek gratification in the sympathy that others show of their plight or condition. While most people do not like the attention others give when they are facing difficult times or situation; there are others are showing. People who bask in the glory of sympathism do not like to make any efforts to change the status of their condition.

For example: If a patient is an illiterate, he will not try to learn and change the status of his illiteracy beacause he likes the sympathy that others show the help that others are willing to render.

18. Intellectualization: By using this mechanism, the intensity of the anxiety is reduced by resorting to a detached, unemotional, intelligent yet abstract language. Mostly used by professionals like doctors, nurses and lecturers.

For example: Providing sex education in a conservative setting. Temporarily separating emotional and cognitive components sometimes helps the individual to deal with parts of an experience when the whole is too much to handle. Over use can leads to boredom.

19. Fantasizing and day dreaming: The motives that cannot be fulfilled in reality are fulfilled by resorting to wishful thinking. Wishful thinking means, thinking as one wishes to. This is done by fantasizing, which means creating a fantasy, unimaginary dream world of one's own. It helps in transporting people to places and events not possible in reality. Sitting in the class and dreaming about the future sometimes the dreams may be full of ambitions which will help as self set standards of achievement. Over use of these may gives to psychological problems.

20. Withdrawal: This is type of coping with some frustrating event in the environment or self by moving away from everyone and everything. It provides temporary relief by giving the person sometime to devise alternate modes of dealing with the problem situation by spending some moments alone. But too much of withdrawal will make the person cut off from reality and out of sync with social world. This mechanism is used by depression clients and also by hypomanics.

IMPLICATION OF DEFENSE MECHANISMS

Advantages

1. If defense mechanisms were not partially successful they would not persist as they do. They give us sometime to solve the problem that might otherwise overpower us. They may provide relief against stress and anxiety until more realistic ways of solving problems are worked out.
2. Mental mechanisms may permit experimentation with new roles and hence teach new modes of adjustment. Even when we adopt new roles for faulty reasons, we expose ourselves to corrective experiences from which we learn. What begins as self-deception may provide occasions for modification of self.
3. Rationalization may actually lead to rational conduct in future because of tendency to search for reasons. The tendency to justify behavior that we have found satisfying may lead to false reasons, but it may also lead to a mere careful analysis of cause-and-effect relationships.
4. Moderate and intellectual use of mental mechanisms, provide a temporary relief to stress and contributes for a healthy living.

Disadvantages

1. Even when behavior based on defense mechanisms is socially useful; it may not prove completely satisfying to the individual as long as the motives underlying the behavior remain so. Actions based on such defense mechanisms never reach their goals, the drive continues and the resulting behavior is not fully stress free.
2. A person's motives or emotions may be so strongly involved that they distort evidence or the problem itself; so that the person is incapable of direct problem solving.
3. Over use and abuse of mental mechanisms give rise to psychological disorders.

Personal and Social Adjustments

For successful living, man has to adjust to himself and his surrounding. Most of the activities of an individual are adjustment to his vocational, social and financial problems. To adjust with different situations is the very nature of man. As man wants to lead a problem and stress free, satisfied and happy life, he tries to adjust with his environment all the time.

According to physiologists, adjustment is an interaction between the environment and organic factors. But according to psychologists, it has a broad meaning. Due to stress and hassles of society upon an individual, he shows his own reactions to the environment. Those reactions may be physical or psychological but keeps balance between individual and his surrounding. This is known as adjustment. The environmental and social pressure may be external or may come from within a man.

For example: In the family a child is allowed to do some work and prohibited to do some other work. He has to stick to certain principles. As interaction taken place between his personal nature and demands of surrounding, from which his personality flourishes. On the other hand there are internal impulses such as hunger, sleep, breathing which control our personality to a great extent. When the internal forces and external forces work in opposite direction, adjustment process becomes complicated. While satisfying our urge, the other unsatisfied impulses create reaction. In such a case mental and physical balance is missed and the individual suffers from frustration.

Good adjustment is constructive and coping with the environment. According to Coleman, by adjustment man makes himself free from mental tension and fulfils his requirements. Again he is capable to establish positive relation with his environment. Smith views that a good adjustment is practical and provides satisfaction. It minimizes frustration and tension for the future. But this does not mean that well adjusted individual does not experience stress or frustration in his life. He also becomes unable and sometimes fails to fulfill all the requirements and reach his goal. He also accepts defeats and frustrations in his life. But as he is capable of facing these problems, his physical and mental balance is not altered. Every person encounters his frustrations in his own ways. So way differ from person to person.

Adjustment Process

Adjustment process starts at womb. At the time of birth, the child is fully dependent on care takers. His requirements are fulfilled by the members of his family and society. His environment seems to him mysterious as a spider's nest. All the persons and objects around him seems to be alike. But gradually when he becomes older he applies his power of perception, sensation and conception and gains better knowledge about his surrounding. Then the child starts thinking about each and every matter he comes across. Development in thinking process leads him to abstract thinking by which he can know about nonexisting things.

At times the child is faced with such situations when his inner and outer requirements work in opposite direction. In such conditions he faces problems. If he solves these problems in a socially approved way his power of adjustment can be said to be well developed. But on the contrary, if he solves them in an illegal and unethical way that shows this mental imbalance.

Stress is the cause for which the individual fails to adjust properly. All the activities of the individual is directed towards a goal. To actualize that goal he applies all his physical and mental energy. If due to any reason he fails to fulfill his ambitions a storm is created in him. This results in tension and loss of physical and mental balance. Man tries in many ways not to let this balance be missed.

The famous psychologist Piaget (1957) conducted a research study on adjustment process. He observed that there are some persons who are bound to their purpose so boldly that in spite of any change or reverse in environment they are not ready to be detached from their goal. There are some other persons who change their aim and objective in tune with the change in the environment. Not only they change their goals but also their behaviors and activities also undergo changes. A positive attitude is required for an effective adjustment.

At birth, the infant's home environment plays an important role in building personal and social adjustments. It is here that the foundations for later social behavior and attitudes are laid. The type of behavior infants show in social situations affects their personal and social adjustments.

By the end of three years, cooperative play and group activities begin to develop and increase in both frequency and duration as the child's opportunities for play with others. Usually children like to play themselves. When they are angry they tend to destroy anything within their reach. Young children learn from others. Generosity replaces selfishness young children, who find satisfaction from warm, close, personal associations with others, gradually attach their affection to people outside the home such as teachers and neighbores. Usually, the same age group children are selected and tries to play with them. Parents encouragement helps to develop otherwise they may fail to play independently. Acceptances, affection and achievement of goals are fulfilled. The search for identity begins later. To achieve a sense of identity, children have an inner assurance that they are able to function independently.

During adolescence, the major social adjustment is towards the member of opposite gender. New social relationships, peer group, values and ethics plays in selection of leaders. Social behavior characterized by cooperativeness responsibility, resourcefullness, interest in others, tact and good manners contribute to acceptance of the adolescent in the social world. Personal traits that contribute to good social adjustments include truthfulness, sincerity, unselfishness and extroversion. Social behavior like teasing, showing off, bossism, uncooperativeness and lack of tact result in rejection by others. The personality traits like selfishness, nervousness, stubbornness, etc. irritate the people. In adulthood, success is seen on their self-concepts and individual personalities.

During middle adulthood, personal adjustments mainly include sexual changes, in men and women, personality changes, physical changes, retirement changes, loss of spouse and also changes in interests. On the social front, middle aged people may enjoy social circle by joining clubs and peer-group and get together parties. These activities reach their peak in late forties and early fifties and then begin to decline as the individual nears to sixties. A descrease in energy and time makes individuals to stay out of circle. Good health and wealth helps to enjoy life; but it is time of the empty-nest, the time when the children no longer stay under the same roof for various reasons. The success with which men and women adjust to middle age can be assessed by four criteria: achievements, emotional states, effect of the physical and psychological changes on personality and the degree of satisfaction or happiness the middle aged person experiences.

More maladjustment occurs at old age. Physical and mental decline makes them vulnerable. Feeling useless, worthless, depressed, feelings of inferiority and resentment are seen in later life. Good home environment favors the old age for happy living, other wise maladjustment and physio-psychological problems spurts up.

Guidance and Counseling

It is quite possible that the earliest occasion in which humans sought a counselor was when Adam reaped the consequences of his eating the apple in the Garden of Eden. Abundance of evidence suggests that persons throughout the ages have sought the advice and counsel of others believed to possess superior knowledge, insights or experiences. In Mahabharat epic, the Lord Krishna acts as counselor and counsels the Arjuna to fight against his own kins. In the early civilizations, the philosophers, priests or other representatives of the gods were seen in roles-offering advice and counseling. In this new era, teachers, books, specialized educationists are offering advice to the needy to meet their demands.

Guidance is helping a way for approach in distress. Crow and Crow define guidance as it is not direction. It is not the imposition of one's point of view upon another. It is not making decisions for an individual which he should make for himself. It is not carrying the burden of another's life. Rather, guidance is assistance made available by a competent counselor to an individual of any age to help him direct his own life, develop his own point of view, make his own decisions. carry his own burdens.

Hamrin and Erikson define guidance as "that aspect of educational program which is concerned especially with helping the pupil to become adjusted to his present situation and to plan his future in the line with his interests, abilities, and social needs".

Mathewson believes that "guidance is the systematic professional process of helping the individual through education and interpretative procedures to gain a better understanding of his own characteristics and potentialities and to relate himself more satisfactorily to social requirements and opportunities in accord with social and moral values". Traxler consider guidance as a help which enables "each individual to understand his abilities and interests, to develop them as well as possible and to relate them to life-goals, and finally to reach a state of complete and mature self-guidance as a desirable member of the social order".

According to Jones, "Guidance involves personal help given by someone; it is designed to assist a person to decide where he wants to go; what he wants to do or how he can best accomplish his purpose; it assists him to solve problems that arise in his life".

CHARACTERISTICS OF GUIDANCE

i. *It is a process:* It helps every individual to help himself, to recognize and use his inner resources, to get goals, to make plans, to work out his own problems of development.
ii. *It is a continuous process:* It is needed right from early childhood, adolescence, adulthood and even in old age.
iii. Choice and problem are the distinctive concerns of guidance as here the individual's unique world of perceptions interacts with the external order of events in his life context.
iv. It is assistance to the individual in the process of development rather than a direction of that development. The aim is to develop the capacity for self-direction, self guidance and self-improvement through an increased understanding of his problems and his resources as well as limitations to solve the problem.
v. *Guidance is a service meant for all:* It is a regular service which is required at every stage for every student, not only for awkward situations and abnormal students. It is a positive program geared to meet the needs of all students.
vi. *It is both generalized and a specialized service:* It is a generalized service because everyone-teachers, tutors, advisers, parent play a part in the program. It is a specialized service because specially qualified personnel as counselors, psychiatrists, psychologists join hands to help the individual to get out of his problem.

PRINCIPLES OF GUIDANCE

According to Hollis and Hollis, there are eight principles on which any guidance programme operates. The principles are:
i. The dignity of the individual is supreme.
ii. Each individual is different from every other individual.

iii. The primary concern of guidance is the individual in his social setting.
iv. The attitudes and personal perceptions of the individual are the bases on which he acts.
v. The individual generally acts to enhance his perceived self.
vi. The individual has the innate ability to learn and can be helped to make choices that will lead to self direction consistent with social improvement.
vii. The individual needs a continuous guidance process from early childhood to old age.
viii. Each individual may at times need the information and personalized assistance best given by competent professional personnel.

GUIDANCE AND COUNSELING

According to Tolbert, "Guidance.... is the total program or all the activities and services engaged in by an educational institution that are primarily aimed at assisting an individual to make and carry out adequate plans and to achieve satisfactory adjustment in all aspects of his daily life. Guidance is not teaching but it may done by teachers. It is not separate from education but it is an essential part of the total educational program. Guidance is a term which is broader than counseling and which includes counseling as one of its services".

Butler makes a logical separation of the counseling process with two phases called 'adjustive' and 'distributive'. In the adjustive phase, the emphasis is on the social, personal and emotional problems of the individual; in the distributive phase the focus is upon his educational, vocational and occupational problems.

Guidance is not compulsion, prescription, domination, cut and dried planning and regimentation. It is not making decisions for the one 'guided'. It is not advice. It is the child who makes the choice of a course or career, the guidance worker just helps the child make that choice as intelligently and as wisely as possible.

Guidance does not mean pampering the student—it tries to provide a more suitable program for him, out of some which may be easier than the average, while others may be difficult. Efforts are made to provide an especially tailored program for every individual.

BASIC ASSUMPTIONS OF GUIDANCE

There are certain fundamental facts which justify the foundation of the guidance concept:

i. The differences between individuals in native capacity, abilities and interests are significant, that is, every person is a complete individual of his own patterns. Native abilities are not usually specified.
ii. Varied type of educational, vocational and social opportunities are available in the real world out of which the individual has to make a selection.
iii. Individual development and progress can be predicted to a great extent with the help of intelligence, aptitude, interests and achievement tests.

FUNCTIONS OF GUIDANCE

Guidance is adjustive in the sense that it helps the students in making appropriate adjustment to the current situations in the educational institution and occupational world; in the home and the community. Professional and individualized aid is given in making suitable adjustment at problem and choice points. Simultaneously, the adjustive attitude in the spirit of Reinold Niebuhr is to be developed in the individuals.

God grant me the serenity, To accept the things I cannot change, The courage to change the things I can. And the wisdom to know the difference.

Guidance has an orientational function. It orients the students in problems but helps to check their emergence and maladjustments. It contributes to the self-development and self-realization of the student while furthering the welfare of the society. It is thus an important instrument of national development.

SCOPE OF GUIDANCE

As the life is becoming complex day by day, the problems for which expert help is needed are rapidly enhancing. The scope of guidance is extending horizontally too much of the social world, to matters of prestige in occupations, to the broad field of social trends and economic development. Guidance is assuming the responsibility for the individual in every direction—it helps in the selection of educational courses and profitable occupations, in job placement in higher education and training occupational settings, improvement of study skills and occupational skills, maintaince of mental health; counseling regarding personal adjustment problems; identifying the gifted and the backward and helping them achieve the maximum. Educational, vocational, social, personal, moral, physical and even marital problems of individuals are the concerns of guidance. Its scope is indeed vast.

NEED FOR GUIDANCE SERVICE IN EDUCATIONAL INSTITUTIONS

Actually, now, the young generation is facing many challenges to live happily. They are derailing from the ideal path. So, there is an urgent case for introducing and strengthening the guidance service in the educational institutions of our country to meet the varied needs of the students, administration and the educational system for the following reasons:

1. To help in the total development of the pupil.
2. To enable students to make proper choices at various stages of their educational career.
3. To help students choose, prepare for, enter upon and progress in a career.
4. To help the student in vocational development.
5. To help students make the best possible adjustments to the situations in the school as well as in the home.
6. To supplement the efforts of home.
7. To minimize the mismatching between education and employment and help in the efficient use of man-power.
8. To identity and motivate the students from weaker sections of society.
9. To help in checking wastage and stagnation.
10. To identify and help students in need of special help.
11. To ensure the proper utilization of time spent outside the classrooms.
12. To increase the holding power of schools.
13. To make secondary and higher secondary education successful.
14. To minimize the incidence of indiscipline.

Today, as never before, the country needs successful educators, doctors, engineers, lawyers, technicians, craftsmen, farmers, inventors, writers, artists, business executives. It is essential that students in the educational institutions are helped and guided to take up courses suited to their needs and aspirations, interests and aptitudes so that they become efficient workers. For optimum individual, social, and national development, guidance needs to be made a regular and continuous activity woven in the educational fabric. No educational program from the primary to the university stage can be complete without a well-planned, systematic, scientific and comprehensive student guidance service.

NURSING PERCEPTIVES

Nurses have a pivotal role to play in the promotion of mental health. In depth knowledge about use and abuse of defense mechanisms helps to serve the clients better a way. She has to act as a counselor, in lieu of therapists in dealing with the problems of clients.

SUMMARY

- Mental hygiene is a manner of life in which the individual's adjustment to his environment.
- Mental health is a state of well-being associated with happiness, contentment, satisfaction, achievement, optimism or hope.
- Abnormal behavior can be defined as behavior that is statistically rare, is deviant from social norms, causes subjective discomfort, does not allow normal, day-to-day functioning, or causes a person to be dangerous to self or others.
- Mental illness is caused by chemical or structural malfunctions in the nervous system.
- Mental health education and use of mass media helps to reduce the incidence of mental disorders.
- Defense mechanisms are those mechanisms by which our reality is guarded and at the same time implemented by translating our real motives into something that we can handle.
- Guidance is a helping approach to the needy.
- Counseling is one-to-one helping relationship that focuses on a person's growth and adjustment and problem-solving and decision making needs.

REVIEW QUESTIONS

1. Discuss the mental health and mental hygiene in detail.
2. Enumerate the characteristics of a mentally healthy person.
3. Discuss the role of defense mechanisms in mental health.
4. What do you mean by adjustment?
5. Discuss differences between guidance and counseling.
6. Discuss importance of counseling in an educational institution.

Chapter 10

Psychological Assessment and Tests

Attempts to measure differences between the psychological characteristics of individuals can be traced back to 400 BC when Hippocrates attempted to define four basic temperament types each of which could be accounted for by a predominant body fluid (humor), blood-sanguine (optimistic), black bile (melancholic) (depressed), yellow-bile-choleric (irritable) and phlegm-phlegmatic (listless and sluggish). The first attempt to scientifically measure the differences between individual mental abilities was made by Sir Francis Galton in the 19th century who tried to show that the human mind could be systematically mapped into different dimensions. He studied, among other things, how people differed in terms of their ability to discriminate between stimuli and by collating the results he obtained and devised a system which would allow an individual's abilities to be compared to those of others an idea on which we rely heavily today.

From the work of people like Galton and his French contemporary, Binet, a picture of the human mental domain emerged which saw general human ability as being composed of a number of specific abilities a view which is still held today. The basic tenet of testing nowadays is based upon the principle of measuring human mental performance under different conditions and then making comparisons between people. Of course the statistical rigor with which this is done today is much greater than was generally applied in Galton's day. There is a bewildering array of tests available to us measuring anything from hand-eye-coordination to high level cognitive operations such as spatial reasoning.

Measurement refers to the process of assigning numerical to events, objects, etc. according to certain rules. In the process of measurement, numerals are used to represent quantities of the attribute that is to be measured. The purpose of measurement is to produce trustworthy data that can be used in statistical analyses. Assessment means evaluation with respect to some standard. Evaluation involves a process of appraisal of an object or event with reference to some standard, which may be social, cultural or scientific.

Types of Tests

Psychological tests are classified in many ways. These are:

Achievement Test or Aptitude Tests

These tests used in academic settings from preschool to college level. They focus on specific educational attainments rather than on psychological attributes. Aptitude tests tell us about future performance. Achievement tests, measure one's performance after a relatively standardized set of experiences (e.g. college algebra), whereas aptitude tests measure learning from essentially unknown and certainly uncontrolled, learning experiences.

Ability Tests

Ability tests focus on the question of what people do when they are at their best. That is, ability tests are designed to measure capacity or potential rather than actual achievement. Examples of ability tests are tests of intelligence or tests of aptitude.

Personality Tests

An individual's personality includes all the characteristic ways of thinking, feeling or behaving. These tests are designed to reveal personality aspects of an individual. Projective and objective methods are used to assess personality. Projective methods tend to be less structured and involve a greater degree of judgement in scoring and interpretation. Clients have a fairly large degree of latitude in choosing how to respond. Objective methods, on the other hand, are more highly structured, scoring is objective and interpretation involves relatively less subjective judgement. Clients have a limited number of choices in how they respond to the test items.

For example: 16 PF, sixteen personality factor test is one of the commonly used personality test which measures 16 characteristics of personality.

Intelligence Test

These are age specific, individual vs group test, verbal or non-verbal tests or the so called language and performance tests.

For example: The Wechsler abbreviated scale of intelligence test. It is made up of vocabulary, block design, similarities and matrix reasoning subsets. The test yields verbal, performance and full scale IQ scores.

Multiple Aptitude Tests

It is recent development in testing intelligence. These tests cover wider functions than intelligence tests. They differentiate among the individual's special assets and liabilities.

Special Aptitude Tests

These tests are used to test very specific and special measures of sensory ability or speed of finger movement or complex tests of art-appreciation or of aptitude for law, medicine and engineering.

Projective Technique

These tests are used to assess intellectual and nonintellectual aspects of personality. Here, the individual is presented with a relatively unstructured or ambiguous task like a picture inkblot or incomplete sentences which permits a wide variety of interpretations by the subjects. The basic assumption underlying projective tests is that individual's interpretation of the task will project his characteristic mode of responses, his personal motives, emotions and desires. All this helps to understand finer aspects of the individual's personality.

Other way of classifying psychological test is on the basis of its nature and the method of conducting or administering. These are:

a. Individual versus group tests: These tests depends on who are taking the test, either single or groups of pupil.

b. Paper, pencil versus performance tests: These tests are printed forms containing questions or such other items which are to be answered by marking marks with pencil. In performance tests it is required to manipulate objects, pictures, blocks and mechanical apparatus by hands.

c. Pictorial, numerical, spatial, verbal tests: These tests depend on the content of the test.

d. Speed versus power tests: A pure speed test restricts with a time limit and the individual differences depend upon the performance. A pure power test has time limit, long enough to permit everyone to answer all the questions or items.

CHARACTERISTICS OF A GOOD PSYCHOLOGICAL TEST

1. The prime characteristic of a good psychological test is its standardization. It includes reliability and validity of the test.
2. A test must be objective, unbiased and assessed in numerical terms.
3. *Sample and Sampling:* A good psychological test will be very widely representative enough to cover a wide range of individuals of both genders at different age groups.
4. It must be culture free.
5. *Reliability:* A good test should be highly reliable. It means that the test should provide similar results even though different investigators administer it, different people score it, different forms of the test are given and the same person takes the test at two or more different times. Uniform construction makes the test more reliable. Reliability is very essential for a test to be scientific and good. Reliability can be determined by using test-retest method, Alternate form method is Split-half method.

a. Test-retest method: In this method, researchers administer the same measure to a large sample of subjects at different interval of time and then correlation of coefficient is calculated. High correlation indicates high consistency and thus high reliability.

b. Alternate form method: It is modified and improved test-retest method. To eliminate practice effect, an alternate test is administered second time with different items but similar in nature as were in first administered test. High correlation in scores obtained at different interval of time indicates high reliability.

c. Split-half method: Here the test items are divided into two halves and then correlation is calculated between the scores of two halves of test. It is also be divided in center or by separating odd and even items in to two halves. High correlation indicates high reliability.

VALIDITY

A good test should be valid. It means that the test must really measure what it has been designed to measure. It is the degree to which a test correlates with some accepted criterion of the behavior being measured. It is of four types:

a. Concurrent validity
b. Predictive validity
c. Content validity
d. Construct validity.

a. Concurrent validity: Here the scores of test are correlated with already established test.
For example: Correlating scores with Raven's progressive matrices. If the correlation is high it indicates that the newly constructed test measures the same ability as Raven's test.

b. Predictive validity: Predictive validity concerned with the degree to which one set of operations can be substituted for another. Here, there is a measure of the property which is taken to be perfect, the criterion, and we seek to estimate scores on it from scores on another measure the predictor. The term prediction as used here does not imply that we are solely concerned with forecasting a future state of affairs, but merely that we are estimating what a given state of affairs is before we actually know. The state of affairs we predict may occur in the future, it may hold at the present time, or it may have held in the past.

c. Content validity: The content validity of a set of operations refers to the degree to which those operations measure the traits which we wish to measure as judged from the characteristics or content of those operations. We examine a test or other measuring instrument and then, on the basis of our "insight' or "wisdom", judge its validity. The question asked is "To what extent do the operations measure what they are supposed to measure?". The answer is based on entirely upon subjective or "professional" judgment, and the degree of validity is given in verbal terms such as "high", "moderate", or "low".

d. Construct validity: It is a logical analysis, not correlation. When the test is designed to measure a theoretical idea, its validity is judged by the extent to which it confirms to the requirements of theory.

e. Norms: Norms are sets of scores obtained by representative groups of people for whom the test is intended. The scores obtained by these groups provide a basis for interpreting any individual's score. Norms are yet another characteristic of a good test.

PRINCIPLES

Psychological tests are used to assess the individual's traits and differences. The test which is to be used must be scientifically constructed and used judiciously. The following ethical and social aspects of test use includes:

1. The user must be a qualified professional.
2. There should be restricted sale of testing instruments. Tests are not for free sale; their sale is restricted to person who meets certain minimum qualification because they are liable to be misused.
3. Protecting privacy and confidentiality is a major concern.
4. Communication of test results should be meaningful, useful and correctly interpreted.
5. Psychological measurement comprises the measurement of mental processes, traits, habits, emotions, etc. Hence the unit of measurement is not fixed and varies during the process of measurement.
   For example: In measurement of intelligence, there is no fixed unit of measurement because some may measure intelligence on the basis of verbal questions, others may prefer to use some particular task in a specified period.
6. In psychological measurement there is no absolute zero point.
   For example: When a person gets a zero on an aptitude test, it does not mean that he has no aptitude for that thing at all.

The said aptitude is perhaps in such a low level that it is not subjecting itself to the test level.

7. Because there is no absolute zero point in psychological measurement, no prediction can be made with definite accuracy.
8. Psychological measurement is indirect.
   For example: It is not easy to measure confidence directly but it has to be done indirectly by studying the responses given by the person concerned upon some tests constructed for that purpose.
9. In psychological measurement only the sample representing a particular quality or trait can be measured but not the entire population.
10. Maintenance of test security is a paramount concern. The results and scores are kept in secure place and with restricted accessibility.

USES OF TESTS

Psychological tests are used in all aspects of life. For worthful decision making, including selection, recruitment, placement and promotion, training, follow-up and evaluation. In clinical settings, the tests are used by health professionals to diagnose the disease, it's severity and for rehabilitative strategies. A qualified nurse may use the assessment techniques to know how a client is responding to care. All decisions involve for planning and prediction. These are the following uses of tests.

1. Recruitment, selection and promotion: In this new era, selection of personnel in different departments such as educational institutions, defense, railways, industry, etc. are carried out with the help of measurement.

For example: Before recruiting nurses, the hospital administration might ask the nurses to go through a psychological test which may measure their adaptability to the job; attitude or any other matter in concern and similar tests can be used for performance appraisal.

2. Classification: Measurement helps in classification of people.

For example: Clients can be classified into different categories of disturbance and specialized as well as individualized care can be provided.

3. Comparison: Individuals differ in all aspects but can be compared on a single aspect.
For example: IQ tests is administered to find out who's IQ level is more than the other.

4. Guidance and counseling: With the help of psychological tests, we can come to know the people's strengths, weaknesses, merits, demerits, complexes, adjustment problems, etc. so that care can be provided by way of counseling and guidance. Nurses can utilize this in providing care to clients.

5. Education: Variety of psychological tests are used in educational field like achievement tests, aptitude test and personality tests for selection and evaluation, etc.

6. Hospitals: Psychological tests can be used in clinicals to diagnose, prognosis and evaluation of the client. It helps for therapeutic management. Various projective tests like Rorschah, word association test, dream analysis can be helpful. Memory tests and IQ tests are also helpful to find out intelligence level and in further it helps in clinical management.

7. According to Cronback: The use of tests are prediction, diagnosis and research.

8. Research: Research is based on scientific measurement. It may be physical, psychological or educational. Research is the key to discover the new type of relationships between variables and to develop and confirm various theoretical approaches. Psychological tests help in obtaining the data for this purpose. Tests are very useful in research purposes.

INTERPRETATION OF TESTS

According to Goldman (1961), identifies four dimensions of test interpretations:

1. *Descriptive:* Tests are used for descriptive information processing. They are used for comparison.
2. *Genetic:* The test data are interpreted in order to show the "how and why" of the individual's behavior or experience.

3. *Predictive:* Tests are helpful to predict the future by knowing the present test scores.
4. *Evaluative:* Tests are good media for evaluative process. Here, we can interpret, specific suggestions, recommendations or professional guidance can be delivered.

NURSING PERCEPTIVES

Tests are useful indicators of health and illness. A qualified nurse must aware about availability of different tests and its uses. She has to encourage the clients to take the tests which in turn help for quality planning and care. Nurse should know in depth about tests, its administration and uses, which contributes for evidence based practice.

SUMMARY POINTS

- Measurement is the process of assigning "numbers to objects (or events or situations) in accord with some rule.
- Assessment involves evaluation with respect to some standard.
- Psychological tests include both projective and nonprojective.
- A test must be standardized. It must have high reliability and validity and must show generalization of scores.
- Psychological tests are used in industry, education, defense and in administrative setting for various reasons.
- A sound knowledge of tests helps the nurse to deliver a quality of care.
- Tests are used for description, prediction and evaluation.

REVIEW QUESTIONS

1. Define test. Briefly discuss the history of measurement.
2. Enumerate the different psychological tests.
3. What is reliability?
4. Explain the characteristics of a good test.
5. What do you mean by validity?
6. Enumerate the uses of tests.

Index

READER'S OPINION

Dear Readers,

Kindly reply to the following request.

1. Do you feel all the units are covered appropriately?
   Yes ……………………..
   No ……………………..

2. Did you have any difficulty to understand the language?
   Unit No.
   Chapter No.
   If Yes Page No.
   Content of para:

3. Do you feel the contents of material is enough to achieve the objectives?
   Yes ………………………..
   No ………………………… Give reasons ……………………..

4. Did the review questions help in testing units?
   Yes ……………………..
   No ……………………..

5. Would you like to add anything in the content of this book.

6. Any other suggestions………………………………..

Students are requested to fill-up this form and send it at the following address:

RAJESH G KONNUR
Professor and Vice Principal
Sri Guru Ram Das College of Nursing
Vallah, Amritsar
Punjab, India